MW00744328

GUTS

GET UNCOMFORTABLE
TO SUCCEED

**EMBRACING
HEALTH,
BALANCE AND
ABUNDANCE**

BETTY FRANKLIN, RN

*Let It Begin with Me
Health Promotions*

Copyright © 2012 by Betty Franklin

All rights reserved. No part of this book may be reproduced by any
mechanical, photographic, or electronic process or in the form of
phonographic recording; nor may it be stored in a retrieval system,
transmitted, or otherwise copied for public or private use without
the prior written permission of the publisher and author.

Every reasonable effort has been made to locate and acknowledge
the owners of copyright material reproduced in this book. The
publisher and author welcome any information regarding errors or
omissions and will gladly address them in subsequent editions.

Cataloguing data available from Library and Archives Canada.

ISBN 978-0-9879102-0-2

Issued also in electronic form.

Design and layout by Kim Monteforte, WeMakeBooks.ca
Cover design by Campbell Walker, Chronic Design
Edited by Andrea Lemieux
Index by Judith Brand
Illustrations by Alex Diochon

Let It Begin with Me Health Promotions
998 Fredonia Drive
Mississauga, Ontario
Canada
L5C 2W4
www.letitbeginwithme.ca

The information in this book is not intended as a substitute for
medical or professional advice. It is strictly the opinion of the
author. It is recommended that you consult with your professional
healthcare provider if you have any acute physical, mental or
emotional health concerns.

Printed and bound in Canada

Dedication

I dedicate this book to the patients I have cared for, the nurses and other healthcare professionals I have worked with and all whom I have crossed paths with. This book would not have been possible without the love and support of my family, my friends and my God.

CONTENTS

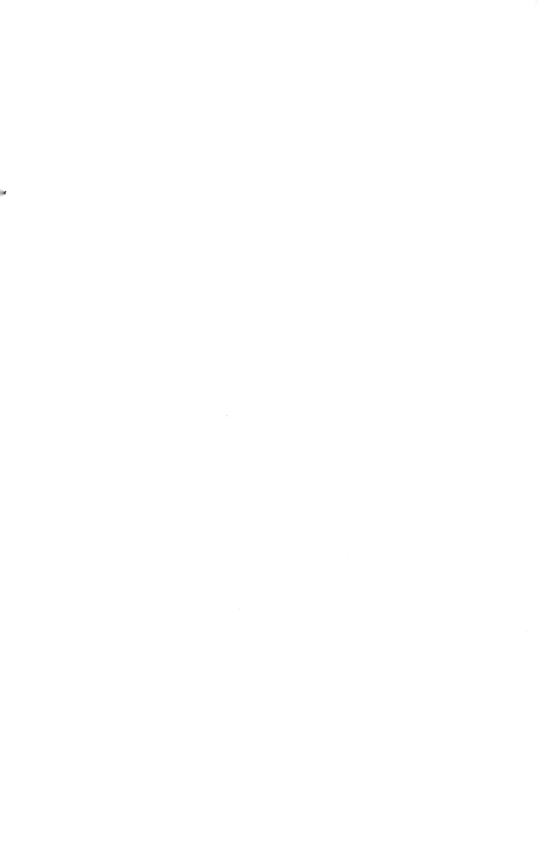

ACKNOWLEDGMENTS

The idea of writing a book first came to me in 2007. And since then, I talked about it with many people, but it was not until someone said to me, "Betty, where's the book?" that I focused on its completion. I had already taken a short course on writing, but still, not much was on paper.

As I became serious about writing the book, I received help and encouragement from many amazing people. This book would not have been possible without their input, support and kind words. It is with heartfelt gratitude that I thank all the people who played a part in developing the concepts, tone and style that led to the completion of this book.

First and foremost, this book would not have been written if not for the many people whom I have cared for throughout my nursing career. Helping others gave me a purpose and passion for their welfare. I thank all those I've had the opportunity and privilege to care for during my career.

To my healthcare colleagues, thank you for the knowledge, expertise and warmth you shared with me, which not only enhanced my career but also opened my eyes to the dedication and commitment you give to your chosen profession. I express my deepest gratitude to all I have worked with.

To the numerous authors, researchers and wise sages whose research, conclusions and beliefs have informed mine and added value and validity to this book, thank you.

To Heidy Lawrance of We Make Books and Kim Monteforte, my designer; Cam Walker, my cover artist; Judith Brand, my indexer; and Alex Diochon, my illustrator, thank you all for your guidance and expertise.

To my editor, Andrea Lemieux, who spent numerous hours editing the manuscript of this new author. Your guidance and expertise have enhanced this book's message immensely. I cannot thank you enough. You have been amazing.

To my friends and family members, who graciously accepted my request to read this book before it went through its final editing, I am forever indebted. You shed light on my writing style, challenged my thinking and pointed out areas that needed improvement and those that needed to be omitted. I am thankful for the commitment each of you gave to my special project. To Peggy Crane, Betty Franklin (my mother-in-law), Colleen Franklin, Doris Grant, Sue Grinyer, Kris Hansen, Eric Izzard, Christine Karcza, Heather Kuurstra, Annika Laale, Kersten London, Mandi Luis-Buckner and Kathy McAndrew, I extend my deepest gratitude.

To all my friends and family, you have added ideas and challenged my thoughts as you listened to me talk about the book for upwards of five years: Helen and Bruce Amey, Sue Atkinson, Jackie Ball, Karen Beaulieu, Leslie Ann Bent, Sandy Breininger, Cameron Clark, Patricia Copeland, Cher Cunningham, Kelly DeBlois, Gail Deere, Sue Douglas, Linda and Peter Hughes, Dawn James, Jill King, Linda Ladd, Pam McLachlan, Wendy and Dave McCleary, Heather McClellan, Paul Nazareth, Donna Pounder, Marianne Rukavina, Susan Train and Cathy Wild, along with everyone in the Franklin and VanderDoelen families. Thank you for your support, time and words of encouragement. Thank you for being a part of my life. I send you all a big hug.

To my children, Nick, Katie and Lucas, and my daughter-in-law, Tracy, thank you for your support and patience while I experimented on you with my ideas, acronyms and short verses. I love you.

This book and these acknowledgments would not be complete without thanking my husband, Scott. You have been with me every step of the way, offering your support, ideas and love. Writing this book progressed more smoothly with you by my side. Thank you.

INTRODUCTION

My healthcare career began in 1975, when I worked part time as a nurses' assistant while studying to become a registered nurse. Ever since, my nursing positions have been on the frontlines. I've worked in a large metropolitan teaching hospital, a large urban hospital and a small community hospital; I have cared for newborns, children, adults and seniors in chronic and acute-care environments. I've also held positions in homecare, private-duty and nursing-home settings.

Throughout the years, I often struggled with the limits to my ability to help those I cared for and served. I would dispense medications and treatments and insert intravenous lines and other tubes. I prepared my patients for surgery, encouraging and supporting them and their families. I dressed patients' wounds, monitored their test results and vital signs and managed the machines attached to them. When their conditions worsened, I responded quickly and worked effectively with the team to stabilize them. I was a member of a large interdisciplinary team. Throughout my work day, I would gently encourage my patients to move and walk about. I fed them and assisted with their personal care. I offered compassion, understanding and health education, rejoicing when they became well enough to go home and saddened when their bodies could no longer sustain them. I made a difference, but it didn't seem to be enough.

During that time, there were amazing advancements in the way disease and illness were diagnosed and treated, and how patients were cared for. These advancements also made a difference, but it still did not seem to be enough.

There were times I became frustrated, cynical and even burned out from the frontline work. Because of this, I began to move my career into other areas. In 1988, I sold homes for two years as a licensed real estate agent. In 2001, after returning to school, I received a diploma that qualified me to work in the not-for-profit sector as a professional fundraiser. And in 2004, I opened a business through which I developed and delivered workshops to promote healthful living.

During these times of transition and learning, I maintained my license and continued to work part time as a registered nurse, always finding it difficult to pull completely away from the field of healthcare and working with people. For me, it is a privilege to help and serve others, and it feels good. I took pleasure in the learning, challenges and diverse groups of people I met. In caring for all kinds of people within the healthcare sector, I've seen life and health renewed and been pleased when people were able to continue living their lives. But I have also seen life and health taken away, and I was disheartened when people's lives ended prematurely. My career as a nurse has given me insight and added color to my life, as well as a sense of purpose.

It is with that insight, color and sense of purpose that I have written this book. It's not a book about the people I've cared for or the different experiences I've encountered. It is about living healthfully within certain key components of life. It's about overcoming and managing the stresses that have been identified as leading to illness. I have written this book to facilitate a better understanding of what healthy looks like, to encourage people to become more sensitive to the choices they make and to urge them to make better choices so they live their lives well.

The concepts and practical guidelines presented in this book are rooted in principles that have stood the test of time. They come from my nursing education and career, personal experiences and the experiences of my patients, family and friends. They come from literature, ongoing education and my constant desire to learn how to live life well, even with its trials and tribulations.

Despite society's continued efforts to find the cause and cure for disease and to improve our health, people still fail in the execution of living truly healthy lives. We continue to live in a world with increasing chronic disease and diminished health. People seem to be sicker, coming to the healthcare system with two or more coexisting medical conditions over and above their initial ailment and diagnosis. With all the advances in healthcare, this has not made sense to me, and I have wondered why this is so. I often asked why we are not living healthier lives with less disease.

Healthcare professionals are very efficient at treating symptoms. The use of medications, tests, treatments and surgeries facilitate improved health and longer lives. Yet these methods have become a cycle that has grown more complicated and expensive.

I have wondered if, by focusing on these methods, we are truly treating the whole person. Is a truly holistic approach being used to care for people and prevent disease?

Do we seek to understand what is happening in peoples' lives— what they are dealing with and what they are thinking? Are we fully aware of the coping strategies they use to address the stress in their lives? Do people manage these concerns in a healthful and holistic manner? I wonder if people are even aware of how the many aspects of their lives influence the way their bodies respond.

To promote health and prevent disease, we must address our basic human needs. We must view people through a lens that encompasses the whole person with their many parts. We must care for them holistically. All facets of our lives and health must be cared for and balanced to maintain our health, prevent setbacks and allow us to live well. To be holistically well, we must care for our physical, mental, emotional, personal and spiritual lives.

The health-promotion workshops I developed and delivered in 2004 were my attempt to create awareness about holistic health and living life well. The participants were interested in the material I presented, and I opened their minds to what holistic living looks like.

The workshops increased their understanding of how their lifestyle choices impact their health. Their desire to improve their lives and the situations they were in increased. I provided them with concepts and tools to guide them toward health and living a balanced life. This book builds on the information and tools I researched, created and presented in those workshops.

This book does not offer remedies for illness and disease. It focuses on promoting health and well-being, and because of this, it is also about preventing disease. Its focal point is helping people understand health and life as a whole with many parts—to understand how different aspects of their health and lives are connected to, and impact, one another. It then offers tools and helpful tips that people may choose to incorporate into their lives.

The concepts I present are founded on holistic health. They are based on the theories and teachings of Dr. Abraham Maslow, a doctor of psychology, and Dr. Hans Selye, an endocrinologist. Maslow's work addressed human needs, and Selye's work addressed stress, disease and the mind-body connection. I also highlight the findings and teachings of Carolyn Myss, a medical intuitive working in the fields of energy medicine and human consciousness. Her work encompasses the thought that our life stories impact our health. She coined the phrase *your biography becomes your biology*.

Combining the points of view of these three experts and my many years of nursing experience, I introduce key components of life and health, which I call the **Six F's of Health and Well-Being**: **F**aith, **F**amily, **F**itness, **F**riends, **F**inance and **F**un. I expand on each of these in the chapters that follow, presenting a range of topics, along with ways to enhance health and find balance, within these components.

Although I am not an authority on any of these areas, and there are many qualified professionals who specialize in them, I offer the experience and knowledge that I have gained from research and study. My intent is simply to create awareness of these components and their impact on your health, and then encourage you to improve your health and life within them.

In support of the **KISS** principle, **K**eep **I**t **S**uper **S**imple, I endeavor to keep the explanation of concepts and ideas in this book uncomplicated. Because our lives and our health can be complex and confusing, I use acronyms to help keep the accompanying principles and practices light and fun. Being short and to the point, these acronyms are also easy to remember.

Interspersed with the acronyms are quotes from many wise, knowledgeable and accomplished individuals. I combine these learning tools with research studies to corroborate the concepts I present.

I also supply **TIP**s **T**o **I**mprove your **P**erformance in life and **ABC**s to offer **A B**etter **C**hoice. As you begin to use these, you will realize it takes **LOVE**, **L**istening and **L**earning, **O**verlooking, **V**alidating and **V**aluing and **E**ffort and **E**nergy, as well as **GUTS**, to live truly healthy lives. Each of us must be persistent, act in love and **G**et **U**ncomfortable **T**o **S**ucceed if we are to live healthfully.

As you read on, I ask you to remain aware that the writing of this book has not been a simple process for me. I am a nurse, not a writer. I learned how to write a book by writing this book. I attended a writing course and read books on how to write. My editor and I, along with my husband, have gone through more edits than we dare to count. To ensure these thoughts and concepts were introduced and presented in a logical and easy-to-follow manner, thirteen friends, family members and colleagues graciously accepted my request to read a full draft before the final edits were completed.

When you become more aware of your current level of health and well-being and become more in tune with how you are living, I hope you will make adjustments and changes to ensure you live life well. I have seen many people die before their time. Many made daily choices they did not know would negatively impact their lives and health in the years to come. Many were either afraid to improve their lives, did not know how or did not have the desire. I hope you live a long, contented and productive life as you persevere in experiencing the richness of life and seek to become all you can be.

Even though I have written a book about balanced, healthful living, I'm aware that my own life and the choices I make are not always healthful, nor are they always balanced. There are days I do well and days I do not. I do, however, routinely ask what I can do to improve myself, my health and my life. Then I endeavor to make the necessary changes. I tell myself to let the change be initiated by me. In doing so, I learn, grow and make better choices.

I've come to realize that if I want to experience and enjoy the wonders of life, the best way to do so is by persistently taking action steps to improve myself. For me to embrace health, balance and abundance, I know I will need to **G**et **U**ncomfortable **T**o **S**ucceed as I ...

Let It Begin with Me!

Chapter 1

UNDERSTANDING HEALTH

What Is Holistic Health?

I believe we all want to live a good life. We desire health and well-being for ourselves, our families and our friends. But we do not always know how to obtain it. Nor do we fully understand what good health and well-being look like.

Webster's dictionary describes *health* as "the condition of being sound in body, mind, or spirit; *esp*: freedom from physical disease or pain." *Well-being* is defined as "the state of being happy, healthy, or prosperous."

Well-being is more than physical health. It is about balance in all areas of our lives. I believe we are well when we have peace of mind in ourselves and in regard to our families and finances. We are well when we have time to pursue what matters most in our lives and can lend a hand to others.

How many of us have such health and well-being? Do you have peace of mind in yourself and regarding your family and finances?

Are you pursuing what matters most to you, or are you stressed, struggling to get through each new day and challenge?

Holism is the functional relationship between parts and wholes. Holistic health describes the health we have within all parts of our being. Along with our physical health, I believe it also includes our thoughts and emotions and the relationship we have with ourselves, others and a higher spirit. It includes how we respond to life's challenges and stresses. It even includes how we manage money. To be healthy from a holistic perspective, we need to have balance within and between each area.

> *"To know balance is to know peace."*
>
> — Dr. Anne Wilson Schaef, American psychotherapist and author

Webster's describes *balance* as "a physical equilibrium; mental and emotional steadiness; equipoise between contrasting, opposing, or interacting elements; to bring into harmony or proportion."

When our lives are not in balance, it is difficult to feel completely well. Like a car with a flat tire, an unbalanced life will not move along well. It begins to wobble from lack of steadiness or equilibrium. Life becomes challenged and stressed. With an understanding of the components of holistic health, we can make better choices to live healthy, balanced and abundant lives.

In chapter 3, I begin to describe each of the **Six F's**, **F**aith, **F**amily, **F**itness, **F**riends, **F**inance and **F**un, and how these components relate to holistic health. First, I'll explain the foundational roots behind these elements through my understanding of the work of Dr. Abraham Maslow, Dr. Hans Selye and Carolyn Myss.

Our Human Needs

Every one of us is motivated by needs. Dr. Abraham Maslow (1908–1970), focused his studies on human potential and motivation. Even though he delivered his theories in the 1940s and 50s, they remain fundamentally sound today, still playing an important role in business, education, social welfare and healthcare. His needs-oriented approach illustrates how seeing the whole picture can be applied to all areas of our lives.

Maslow arranged his list of human needs in a hierarchical format according to what he believed to be important for human survival and for their power to motivate. Beginning with our basic needs, he theorized that we do not move to satisfying our next need until the previous one is met. He identifies the six human needs as follows:

1. Physiological: Our need for air, water, food, shelter and clothing
2. Security: Our need for a safe and secure environment in which to live
3. Social: Our need for love, acceptance and belonging
4. Self-esteem: Our need to be valued—regarding personal worth, self-respect and respect from others

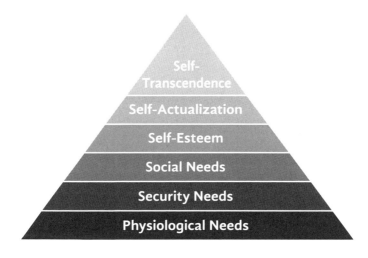

Maslow's Hierarchy of Needs

5. Self-actualization: Our need for personal growth and interest in fulfilling our potential—our need to be and do what we are born to do

6. Self-transcendence: Our need to find higher meaning in life

Humans are emotional, spiritual and feeling creatures. We need to feel safe and secure physically, mentally and emotionally. We need to grow, be productive, love and be loved. We need to participate in life in a way that is meaningful and gives us purpose.

In Western society today, most of us have our physiological needs met. We may struggle with the need for safety and security, when employment opportunities and safe neighborhoods and homes are compromised. Family and relationship problems, job changes, financial turmoil, death and other disruptive life transitions can also compromise our need for safety and belonging. This, in turn, can lower our self-esteem and self-worth, as well as our need to be the best we can be.

Generally, we put greater emphasis on meeting our physical and material needs than meeting other human needs. We also do not address the impact that the stress of not meeting these other needs has on our health and well-being.

Stress and Balance

Dr. Hans Selye (1907–1982), was one of the early pioneers in the study of stress and disease and the mind-body connection. He described three stages the body goes through when we adapt to a stressful event.

1. Alarm: When the body senses stress, the central nervous system is aroused, mobilizing the *fight-or-flight response*. Some call this the *adrenaline rush*. The heart rate and blood pressure increase. Breathing becomes faster. Metabolism and mental activity increase.

2. Resistance: Using physiological resources, the body attempts to adapt to the challenging situation and return to a homeostatic state.

3. Exhaustion: When the challenging situation lasts too long, the body's resources are depleted and can no longer produce needed hormones. The immune system is impaired, organ damage occurs and illness sets in.[1]

The body strives to sustain a steady state of internal balance, called *homeostasis*. To be and stay healthy involves a dynamic process of successfully adapting to stresses and maintaining biological stability in the midst of ever-changing situations and conditions.

Every cell in the body is involved in maintaining homeostasis. Cells are our basic building blocks. They are minute portions of living substance that create and renew all parts of the body. Groups of cells come together to form organs, tissues, bones and more. The body has more than fifty trillion cells, each working independently to sustain our lives and health. Each individual cell is specifically adapted to perform a particular function. For example, red blood cells perform the function of transporting oxygen from our lungs to other cells.

In all cells, oxygen combines with carbohydrates, fats or proteins to release the energy required to function. The way nutrients are changed into energy does not vary from cell to cell. All cells discard the waste generated from the chemical production of this energy into the fluids that surround them. Cells are like small chemical factories, combining and separating various elements to create energy. Rebecca Skloot, an award-winning science writer, explains how our cells are crammed full of molecules and vessels, endlessly shuttling enzymes from one cell to another and pumping water, nutrients and oxygen in and out of the cells. They work 24/7, cranking out sugars, fats, proteins and energy to keep us running. Our cells continually grow and divide. They get their jobs done, whether controlling your heart-

1. Hans Selye, *The Stress of Life* (New York: McGraw-Hill, 1956), 324.

beat or helping your brain understand the words on this page. With cell division, known as *mitosis*, embryos grow into new babies and the body constantly creates new cells for healing wounds or replenishing blood that may have been lost. Skloot calls it "a perfectly choreographed dance."[2]

Every year the body produces trillions of new cells to replace those that have worn out. Whenever cells are destroyed, the remaining cells divide again and again until the need to replenish them has been met. We cannot exist without the constant reproduction of cells. It keeps us internally balanced and our bodies in a homeostatic state.

When this balanced interaction of cells is disrupted, it impacts our health and well-being. Stress disrupts this balance. Whether it's an injury, lack of nutrients, an invasion of parasites or life challenges, stress impacts the body's homeostasis. When stress occurs, the body responds in one of two ways: It adapts successfully or it fails to adapt.

Controlled by the nervous and endocrine systems, the stress response redirects energy to the organ that is most affected by the stress. If the body adapts well to stress, it recovers, returning to a balanced or homeostatic state. If it fails to adapt, the body continues to function at an increased rate and exhaustion sets in. Stress speeds up the body's internal responses.

Picture someone spinning their wheels, going round and round, trying to maintain their balance while dealing with life's trials and challenges, struggling, exhausted and losing their balance. As the wheel spins

---

2. Rebecca Skloot, *The Immortal Life of Henrietta Lacks* (New York: Crown Publishers, 2010), 3.

faster and faster, their body tires from the continuous release of epinephrine (adrenaline) that speeds up their internal functions. If brakes are not properly activated to slow them down, in time they will begin to wobble. They may break down, spin off their axis or crash.

The body, like the person in the spinning wheel, can maintain a fast pace for only so long. Stress impacts the body at the cellular level. When we do not adapt well, we continue to function at an increased rate and exhaustion sets in. Homeostasis is disrupted. There's no peace or balance. Illness and disease set in. Not a nice picture.

The fight-or-flight response initiated by stressful situations is appropriate when we must respond quickly to an event that requires an immediate response. But remember, when stress continues for long periods of time, the increased heart rate, blood pressure, respirations, metabolism and mental activity brought on by the fight-or-flight response are not healthful.

As physical or psychological stressors cause increased activity inside our cells and bodies, certain symptoms present themselves externally. A person dealing with stress may

- always be in a hurry;
- be unable to concentrate;
- be irritable;
- clench their fists or jaw;
- experience loss of appetite or increased appetite;
- cry, yell or have mood shifts;

- smoke or drink excessively;
- overeat, gamble or use drugs;
- lose their of sense of humor, self-esteem or sexual desire; or
- feel lonely, anxious or depressed.

In time, as stressful situations continue unabated, the organ damage caused by the nonstop acceleration of the body's systems leads to discomfort, cell damage and sickness. Most sicknesses follow a typical pattern of symptoms called *pathogenesis*, which are influenced by the following:

- Genetic factors: Our tendency toward obesity, heart disease or bowel problems
- Unhealthful behaviors: Smoking, using drugs, overeating and not exercising
- Attitudes and personality type: Acceptance, denial, anger and type A personality
- Perceptions of health and disease: Fear, worry and anxiety

Positive and negative situations in our lives stress the body, affecting us physically, mentally, emotionally and behaviorally. Dr. Richard Brown, associate professor of clinical psychiatry at the University of Columbia, states, "We now believe that 80 percent of illness is stress related, that whatever your genetic weak link is, stress will trigger it."[3] Did you know that

- seventy-five to ninety percent of doctor office visits are for stress-related ailments or complaints;
- stress is linked to the six leading causes of death: heart disease, cancer, stroke, respiratory disease, accidents and diabetes; and
- the lifetime likelihood of an emotional disorder is more than fifty percent and is often related to chronic, untreated stress reactions?

---

3. Hagar Scher, "Cultivating Calm," *Good Housekeeping* (April 2007): 140.

The manner in which we handle stress plays an important role in our health and well-being. Because change and difficult situations cause us stress, learning to accept and adapt reduces its damage. Genetic factors *plus* unhealthful behavior *plus* personality type *plus* attitude *plus* perception impact not only life but also how healthy we are. The better we are at maintaining internal balance when we deal with stress, the greater our ability to live healthy lives and prevent disease.

When it comes to illness and disease, considering the whole person and how our human needs are or are not being met provides a complete story of what is going on. Understanding what has happened and is happening in our individual lives, as well as how these circumstances affect us emotionally and mentally, are important factors when examining our health from a holistic perspective. Including our stressors, and our responses to them, provides a comprehensive understanding of what influences our health and well-being.

> *"The doctor of the future will give no medicine, but will interest his patients in the care of the human frame, in diet and in the cause and prevention of disease."*
>
> — Thomas Edison (1847–1931), American scientist and inventor

Your Biography Becomes Your Biology

In her book *Anatomy of the Spirit: The Seven Stages of Power and Healing*, Caroline Myss says, "Every second of our lives—and every mental, emotional, creative, physical, and every resting activity with which we fill those seconds—is somehow known and recorded. Every judgment we make is noted. Every attitude we hold is a source of positive or

> *"Every patient carries her or his own doctor inside."*
>
> — Albert Schweitzer (1875–1965), German physician, theologian and philosopher

negative power for which we are accountable." She sums this up by saying, "Your biography becomes your biology." In other words, your life stories and stresses have an effect on your health and well-being.

Stress often occurs when our needs are in jeopardy or are not being met. How do you feel when you are stressed and your needs are unfulfilled? How do you feel when you have an argument with a family member or friend? When faith in yourself is battered? When your finances are threatened? You may feel anger, fear, anxiety or worry. You may feel overwhelmed, frustrated and even become depressed.

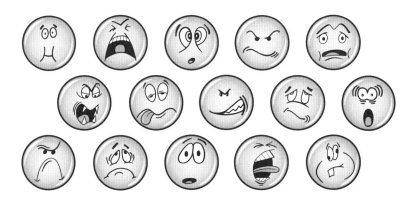

How Do You *Feel When You're Stressed?*

How do you behave? You may be irritable, unable to concentrate or always in a hurry. You may lose your sense of humor. You may eat, drink or smoke in excess.

You may find yourself suffering from a headache, nausea or diarrhea. You may stop taking good care of yourself, causing your resistance to illness to weaken.

Do you tell your healthcare professional about the struggles you have with your family, friends or colleagues? Or do you simply tell them of your insomnia and lack of energy? Do you tell them that you are dealing with low self-esteem? Or do you only mention the sense of physical pain in your joints, chest or back? Do you share details of your financial challenges?

On the other hand, do healthcare professionals ask or know how you manage all your human needs and life challenges?

When Myss, in her role as a medical intuitive, assists doctors to diagnose and treat a patient's symptoms, she incorporates three concepts:

1. Your biography becomes your biology.

2. Personal power is necessary for health.

3. You alone can help yourself heal.

> *"Blessed are the balanced; they shall outlast everyone."*
> — Rick Warren, American author and pastor

Let It Begin with Me!

The teachings of Maslow and Selye and many other researchers, my nursing and life experiences and Myss's concepts together reinforce my belief and understanding that

- our personal history, choices, situations and responses to life's challenges and stresses affect our health and our lives;

- our personal involvement and abilities are necessary components in achieving balanced health and well-being; and

- we are each responsible for ourselves.

These concepts are the basis for this book and the life and health-care programs I deliver.

Getting started and staying the course is not easy. We may know what we need to do, but do not initiate the actions. We may not know what to do, so we remain stuck with what we have become accustomed to. Or we may not have the desire or believe we do not have the time to implement change. But we cannot improve or succeed in living truly healthy and abundantly balanced lives when we are not prepared to do the work. When we do not have the **GUTS** to **G**et **U**ncomfortable **T**o **S**ucceed, we will not succeed, and embracing health, balance and abundance takes **GUTS**.

The introduction to this book and the following chapters end with Let It Begin with Me! When it comes to our health and well-being, this principle is key to discovering and initiating new ways to live well. Let it begin with me is a call to action. It is a proactive rather than a reactive response to healthful living. It states we are no longer willing to wait for something to happen before we take action. It says we are willing to first play our part.

When we begin with ourselves and seek better ways, skills and habits, we begin to take calculated risks. As a statement, it reminds us to be responsible for ourselves. It asks us to change what we can. Our lives and our health improve as we begin to make better choices.

In spite of copious amounts of research and information that result in health-promoting programs and services, many of us, nonetheless, fall short in living truly healthy and fulfilling lives. As I searched for my own answers to why we have such difficulty, I came to believe that in order to live healthy, balanced and abundant lives, we need to begin with ourselves, and we need to manage our health and our stress from a broader, whole-person perspective.

Being aware of our mental, emotional, creative, physical and resting activity assists us in managing our health and stress differently. Healthcare professionals are not aware of, nor do we tend to seek out, this information. We are not aware of all the stresses people encounter and still endure. But you know what has happened in your life. You know your pressure points; you know what causes you tension. You have the ability to know how your mental, emotional, creative, physical and resting activities have affected and still affect you.

Consider the theories of Maslow, Selye and Myss as you read this book. Consider how you and your body respond to injury, stress and life experiences. Consider Dr. Maslow's hierarchy of human needs and Dr. Selye's findings on stress, disease and the mind-body connection. Consider the findings of Caroline Myss. Ask yourself the following:

- Is my biography becoming my biology?
- What personal skills, habits and strengths can I develop to decrease the impact of stress on my life, my family and society?
- What can I do to help myself be a healthy and balanced person?

We all know disease is easier to prevent than to cure. The Let It Begin with Me principle calls for action. It asks us not to wait for something to happen before we take responsibility for our health and well-being. It asks us to build our self-esteem,

> *"Every human being is the author of his own health and disease."*
>
> — Buddha (c. 563–483 BCE), Indian spiritual teacher

develop loving relationships and manage our finances well—to be content and at peace. It calls on us to do our part.

Just as there are many traffic rules to adhere to, whether or not the police are around, there are also many health and lifestyle rules and guidelines to adhere to, but there is no one to enforce rules about health and well-being. It is an individual choice to be or not *be obedient to the unenforceable laws of health and well-being*.

These choices can be anything from learning something new, saying no to fatty foods or changing careers. It can be going for a walk, starting a conversation to create a new friend or saying I'm sorry. It can be speaking less, listening more or sharing your feelings. Whatever it is, it needs to begin with each of us as individuals.

It is said that we use only ten percent of our potential. I believe that means we have nine times more potential to develop, grow and strengthen. We have capabilities we do not know we have and

> *"If we did all the things we are capable of doing, we would literally astonish ourselves."*
>
> — Thomas Edison (1847–1931), American scientist and inventor

potential we fail to give ourselves credit for. We have many skills to learn and opportunities to pursue. We are capable of doing so much more with our lives and so much more for our health.

In order to live healthy, balanced and abundant lives, in order to be the best we can be, each of us needs to be encouraged, motivated and pushed to do and say …

Let It Begin with Me!

Chapter 2

BEING SELF-AWARE

You Are a Magnificent Masterpiece!

Do you ever contemplate the marvel of you—how you were made and how your body and mind function? Consider how your respiratory system works as you breathe; how your heart pumps oxygen-rich blood through your body; and how your nerve endings cause you to feel soft, coarse or sharp objects. Consider how your bones are linked together so you can move, and how your muscles give you strength to help you lift and bend. Consider how amazing you are:

> *"He who knows others is learned; he who knows himself is wise."*
>
> — Lao-Tzu, ancient Chinese philosopher

- Your brain thinks at a rate of 800 words per minute and has over 60,000 thoughts per day.
- Your body consists of 100 trillion cells.
- Your eyes have 100 million receptors.
- Your ears contain 24,000 fibers.

- Your skeleton is composed of 200 bones that are the framework for 500 muscles, 7 miles (11 km) of nerve fiber and 60,000 miles (96,500 km) of blood vessels that lead to a heart that pumps 2,000 gallons (7,500 L) of blood in just one day.

Just think how all your thoughts, cells, receptors, bones, muscles, organs, nerve fibers, blood and vessels work together every second, minute and hour of the day for all the years of your life. You truly are a magnificently masterpiece.

What was the likelihood of your conception? You were conceived by the release of upwards of 500 million sperm and 1,000 eggs. What were the odds? Only one sperm connected with one egg. Once connected, it took close to 280 days for you to develop into an average length of 20 inches (50.8 cm) and weight of 6 to 9 pounds (2.7 to 4 kg) before you were ready to enter the world.

Alexander Tsiaras is an internationally renowned technologist, artist and journalist. He and his company, Anatomical Travelogue, produced a spectacular video based on medical imaging showing the progress of fetal development to birth called *Conception to Birth*.[1] This video gives you an understanding of the wonder of your creation, especially when you consider that at any point during this entire process something could go wrong.

Consider how much you grew and learned in your first year after birth. On average, you doubled your birth weight in six months and tripled it in one year. You learned to roll over, crawl and probably began to walk. You spoke your first words.

Each of us is wonderfully and uniquely made. When you think about this, how can you not be proud of who you are and what you have accomplished? Be aware of your abilities and remind yourself of how much more you can do. But remember, you need to maintain

---

1. Alexander Tsiaras, *Conception to Birth—Visualized*, TED: Ideas Worth Spreading video, 9:38, filmed December 2010, www.ted.com/talks/alexander_tsiaras_conception_to_birth_visualized.html.

your strength and stamina as well as your body's intricate balance and harmony. You need to know that poor nutrition, a sedentary lifestyle and negative thoughts will lead your body to disharmony, imbalance and disease.

The Six F's of Health and Well-Being

Before you consider what more you can accomplish, I would like to share with you how I came to present the topic of balanced, holistic health through the Six F's of Health and Well-Being.

Because we all have needs, I'll begin again with Dr. Abraham Maslow and his hierarchy of human needs. I have taken his hierarchical list and presented them in a circular format with six equal parts to represents holistic health and living.

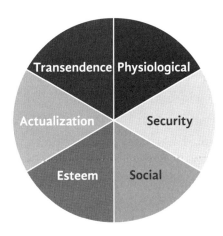

Maslow's Hierarchy of Needs

To express these needs in more practical and simplified terms, I have created a similar circle representing the Six F's of Health and Well-Being.

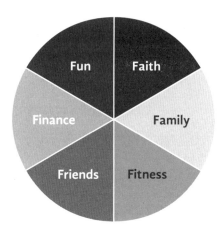

The Six F's of Health and Well-Being

As you read about each of the **Six F's** in the following chapters, you will find that together they encompass all of Maslow's needs. Our physiological needs are addressed within the **F**itness component. Our social and esteem needs are addressed through **F**amily and **F**riends. Security needs, along with our physiological and social needs, are incorporated into **F**inance. The **F**un component addresses both social and esteem needs, whereas one's **F**aith in oneself, others and a higher spirit integrates our need for transcendence or higher meaning, as well as our need for self-actualization and being the best we can be.

The **Six F's** represent the foundational components I believe we need to live healthy and abundantly balanced lives. In the chapters that follow, I delve further into each component, showing how they relate to your health and well-being in the following way:

1. **F**aith: The faith you have in yourself, others, life processes and in a higher spirit

2. **F**amily: Your relationships with your family of origin and your chosen family

3. **F**itness: Your level of physical, nutritional, environmental, mental, emotional and spiritual fitness

4. **F**riends: Your relationships with your buddies and those with whom you work and volunteer

5. **F**inance: Your relationship with money—how much is enough and how to get it, keep it safe, grow it, have fun with it and give it away

6. **F**un: Your attitudes, choices, values and principles and how they impact the fun in your life

Each component influences our ability to live holistically—in homeostasis. To maintain harmony with ourselves, others and the world, we need to learn to balance them. To help you understand more clearly, instead of continuing to represent our needs as pieces of a pie, I also present them in the form of a wheel with six spokes.

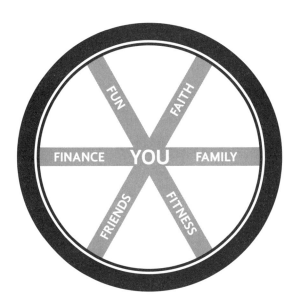

Balance Wheel of Health and Well-Being

When one area of life receives more attention than another, or when we become complacent about our lives, our balance wheels of health and well-being slow down, lose their momentum or become unstable. To live balanced, healthy lives, it is not enough to take care of the parts of life that we enjoy. We need to be aware of, manage, maintain and balance all parts. If we don't, then our "flat" wheels won't roll or move us forward. We can eat healthful food and exercise four times a week, but if we neglect our relationships with family and friends, make no time for rest and fun and compromise our financial stability, we will remain out of balance.

When you have a dispute with a loved one, going for a run or calling a friend can help ease your tension about the situation. But if you do not resolve the situation, your relationship remains tense and stressed. It affects your future communication with each other. Action needs to be taken. You need to settle the disagreement to maintain a strong, loving and respectful rapport. Unhealthy relationships impair your health.

> *"Anytime we are doing too much or too little of something, we are out of balance."*
>
> — Joyce Meyer, American charismatic, author and speaker

If you manage your finances by living paycheck to paycheck, never slowing down your spending to save money, funds needed or wanted to purchase a home, go on vacation or retire in comfort are jeopardized. Unhealthful money habits affect your lifestyle and your health.

When you look at your life from a holistic perspective, with all its components, you see a comprehensive picture. As you develop your awareness of how each component can affect your health, you become aware of your need to change, take positive actions and make better choices.

Is "Normal" Healthy?

In the 1950s and 60s, it was "normal" for people to smoke, but it wasn't good for their health. Today it is normal for servers at restaurants or fast-food outlets to offer us the opportunity to order more food or larger portions. Bigger is better has become the norm, but is it healthful?

It is normal for people to text others while in meetings, at restaurants and in the company of family and friends, but is it a healthful way to build relationships and effective communication skills? It is normal for families not to eat meals together, but is it a way to build healthy, strong and connected family relationships? It is normal for people to buy what they want when they want, but is it healthful for their bank account?

Many people act and respond in a way that has become the norm, but does this normal behavior help us build a healthy mind, body and soul? Changing established patterns, behaviors and responses is difficult. Making the decision to change is like pruning a garden. A garden grows fully and abundantly when it is pruned and the weeds are pulled out.

> *"We can bring ourselves to a place where rushing, high adrenaline, and frantic no longer feel normal or desirable."*
>
> — Dr. Anne Wilson Schaef, American psychotherapist and author

The process of pruning and weeding ourselves of unhealthful behaviors may cause some pain, but it leads to healthier, balanced and more abundant lives. We need to be consistent in pruning, weeding and cultivating our lives. It takes work, time and energy to change our way of living, acting, thinking and believing. It takes **GUTS**, or **G**etting **U**ncomfortable **T**o **S**ucceed.

Learning How to Live

How do you learn how to live? I believe you begin by becoming aware of how you are presently living your life and by understanding what you are living for.

Lifelong learning creates awareness and new knowledge that expands our minds. It helps us grow and acquire new skills. It helps us realize how much we do not know. Learning opens up the world to us; it makes life more exciting, interesting and fulfilling. Through learning we become aware of what is happening around us and of new opportunities to experience.

> *"As long as you live, keep learning how to live."*
>
> — Seneca (4 BCE–CE 65), Roman philosopher, statesman and dramatist

I have a simple exercise for you to do. You will need a pen and paper. To begin, draw a circle. This circle represents all the knowledge in the world. With your pen, take a small piece of pie out of the circle. This piece represents the *knowledge you know you know.* Take out another piece that is just a little larger than the first. This represents *the knowledge you know you do not know.* You will have a circle with two pieces taken out of it. What remains?

All the *knowledge you do not know you do not know* is what remains. And that's a lot of knowledge! The whole pie is known as the *Circle of Knowledge.* In it is a world of new knowledge and information available to you. All you need do is reach out for it.

Sometimes we limit ourselves because we have not taken the time to become aware of ourselves and the world in which we exist. Following are four questions to help you create that awareness. Please take a few moments to complete each question.

1. What aspects of your life make you feel good?

   _____

   _____

   _____

   _____

Others have listed family and friendships; travel, leisure, hobbies, sports and reading; growth, knowledge and experiences; food and entertainment; pets; a long, happy and healthy life; and laughter, joy and contentment.

2. What are the rewards of good health in your life?

_____

_____

_____

_____

_____

Some rewards of good heath include having a feeling of well-being; feeling empowered to do many things; having choices, variety and opportunity; looking good and feeling good; the ability to earn an income; being able to help others; being able to build dreams; and living a long life.

> *"To laugh often and much; to win the respect of intelligent people and the affection of children; to earn the appreciation of honest critics and endure the betrayal of false friends; to appreciate beauty; to find the best in others; to leave the world a bit better, whether by a healthy child, a garden or a redeemed social condition; to know even one life has breathed easier because you have lived. This is to have succeeded."*
>
> — Ralph Waldo Emerson (1803–1882), American essayist, lecturer and poet

3. What does it cost you to live a good life?

_____

_____

_____

_____

Have you considered the costs of taking care of yourself physically, mentally and emotionally; knowing yourself; continual
learning; keeping an open mind; exercising effort, discipline
and commitment; making wise choices guided by sound mor-
als, values and principles; building healthy relationships with
family, friends and colleagues; and managing your finances well?

> *"I think the purpose of life is to be useful, to be responsible, to be honorable, to be compassionate. It is, after all, to matter, to count, to stand for something, to have made some difference that you lived at all."*
>
> — Leo C. Rosten (1908–1997), American teacher, academic and humorist

4. What is the purpose of your life?

_____

_____

_____

_____

_____

Have you heard about the *dash*? The
dash is found on a person's headstone
between the two inscribed dates. It represents the span of a person's life, for example
1921–2011. The dates on the headstone mark the length of
time the person lived, but the real story of their life is contained
within the dash. The dash is about how the years were lived.
The dash includes who the person was, what he or she accomplished and the impact their life made on family, friends,
colleagues, community and the rest of humanity.

Developing Self-Awareness

To assist you in knowing and being aware of yourself and your life, I have two exercises for you to complete. The "I" statement exercise and the balance wheel exercise are based on the **Six F's of Health and Well-Being:** **F**aith, **F**amily, **F**itness, **F**riends, **F**inance and **F**un. When you complete the exercises, you will become more aware of yourself and how you are living your life. You will discover how you can experience each of these components in balance and holistically.

> *"Know thyself."*
>
> — Socrates (469–399 BCE), Greek philosopher

The exercises are intended to create self-awareness and are designed to work together. There are no right or wrong answers as they are about you and your life. To complete the "I" statement exercise, read the affirmations; there are ten "I" statements within each of the six components. As you read each statement, think how it applies to your life. Ask, "How satisfied am I with this aspect of my life?" or "How am I doing in regards to this statement?" Rate your answer on a scale from one to ten, with one representing no satisfaction and ten representing very satisfied.

THE "I" STATEMENT EXERCISE

FAITH: In yourself, in others, in life processes and in a higher spirit	
1. I believe in myself, trust myself and like the person I am.	1 2 3 4 5 6 7 8 9 10
2. I welcome change and know things work themselves out.	1 2 3 4 5 6 7 8 9 10
3. I practice self-discipline and self-control.	1 2 3 4 5 6 7 8 9 10
4. I trust the people in my life.	1 2 3 4 5 6 7 8 9 10

5. I am a positive person.	1 2 3 4 5 6 7 8 9 10
6. I have a dream and goals I am working toward.	1 2 3 4 5 6 7 8 9 10
7. I trust the process of life.	1 2 3 4 5 6 7 8 9 10
8. I know my beliefs affect the choices I make in a positive way.	1 2 3 4 5 6 7 8 9 10
9. I have a spiritual component to my life.	1 2 3 4 5 6 7 8 9 10
10. I do something every day to help me become a better person.	1 2 3 4 5 6 7 8 9 10

FAMILY: Your family of origin, immediate family and/or chosen family	
11. I enjoy time with all my family members.	1 2 3 4 5 6 7 8 9 10
12. I know how to set boundaries in family relationships.	1 2 3 4 5 6 7 8 9 10
13. I teach my children to be self-sufficient and of good character.	1 2 3 4 5 6 7 8 9 10
14. I offer praise regularly to family members.	1 2 3 4 5 6 7 8 9 10
15. I feel accepted and loved by my family members.	1 2 3 4 5 6 7 8 9 10
16. I communicate well with my family members.	1 2 3 4 5 6 7 8 9 10
17. I am committed to playing an active role in the lives of the children in my life.	1 2 3 4 5 6 7 8 9 10
18. I spend quality time with my partner at least twice a week.	1 2 3 4 5 6 7 8 9 10

19. I allow family members to see my vulnerabilities.	1 2 3 4 5 6 7 8 9 10
20. I show my family members that I love them unconditionally.	1 2 3 4 5 6 7 8 9 10

FITNESS: Your level of physical, nutritional, environmental, mental, emotional and spiritual fitness	
21. I am physically active a minimum of thirty minutes three times a week.	1 2 3 4 5 6 7 8 9 10
22. I am involved in creative work, studies or activities consistent with my values.	1 2 3 4 5 6 7 8 9 10
23. I regularly participate in a spiritual practice.	1 2 3 4 5 6 7 8 9 10
24. I manage my time effectively.	1 2 3 4 5 6 7 8 9 10
25. I spend time outdoors appreciating nature.	1 2 3 4 5 6 7 8 9 10
26. I limit my intake of alcohol, nicotine and drugs.	1 2 3 4 5 6 7 8 9 10
27. I set healthful limits for the amount of Internet, social media and TV I engage in.	1 2 3 4 5 6 7 8 9 10
28. I routinely get seven to eight hours of sleep a night.	1 2 3 4 5 6 7 8 9 10
29. I eat five to seven servings of fresh fruits and vegetables every day.	1 2 3 4 5 6 7 8 9 10
30. I understand my feelings and respond to them appropriately.	1 2 3 4 5 6 7 8 9 10

FRIENDS: Your buddies and those with whom you work and volunteer	
31. I have one or more close friends.	1 2 3 4 5 6 7 8 9 10
32. I am involved in service or volunteer work.	1 2 3 4 5 6 7 8 9 10
33. I enjoy the people I meet.	1 2 3 4 5 6 7 8 9 10
34. I know how to be my own best friend.	1 2 3 4 5 6 7 8 9 10
35. I enjoy a satisfying social life.	1 2 3 4 5 6 7 8 9 10
36. I have friends who respect my values.	1 2 3 4 5 6 7 8 9 10
37. I know how to set boundaries with my friends.	1 2 3 4 5 6 7 8 9 10
38. I offer help and assistance to others.	1 2 3 4 5 6 7 8 9 10
39. I handle conflict with others in a healthful manner.	1 2 3 4 5 6 7 8 9 10
40. I enjoy the work I do.	1 2 3 4 5 6 7 8 9 10

FINANCE: Your relationship with money—how much is enough and how to get it, keep it safe, grow it, have fun with it and give it away	
41. I earn the money I need to meet my financial obligations.	1 2 3 4 5 6 7 8 9 10
42. I earn the money I believe I deserve.	1 2 3 4 5 6 7 8 9 10
43. I spend money on what I need rather than on what I want.	1 2 3 4 5 6 7 8 9 10
44. I have financial assets/equity to build on.	1 2 3 4 5 6 7 8 9 10
45. I have a savings and investment plan I follow and review regularly.	1 2 3 4 5 6 7 8 9 10
46. I ask for help to plan my financial future.	1 2 3 4 5 6 7 8 9 10
47. I have an up-to-date will.	1 2 3 4 5 6 7 8 9 10

48. I donate money to a charitable cause I believe in.	1 2 3 4 5 6 7 8 9 10
49. I teach and encourage my children to earn and wisely manage their own money.	1 2 3 4 5 6 7 8 9 10
50. I take time to enjoy and have fun with some of the money I earn.	1 2 3 4 5 6 7 8 9 10

FUN: Your attitudes, choices, values and principles and how they impact the fun in your life	
51. I know how to say and use the word *no*.	1 2 3 4 5 6 7 8 9 10
52. I have respect for and abide by the law.	1 2 3 4 5 6 7 8 9 10
53. I laugh easily and regularly take part in fun and enjoyable activities.	1 2 3 4 5 6 7 8 9 10
54. I have someone to whom I stay accountable.	1 2 3 4 5 6 7 8 9 10
55. I look honestly at myself and admit to my foibles and weaknesses.	1 2 3 4 5 6 7 8 9 10
56. I seek advice and support from others.	1 2 3 4 5 6 7 8 9 10
57. I forgive myself and others.	1 2 3 4 5 6 7 8 9 10
58. I make wise choices according to my values and principles.	1 2 3 4 5 6 7 8 9 10
59. I am grateful for all I have in my life.	1 2 3 4 5 6 7 8 9 10
60. I strive for peace and calmness of mind.	1 2 3 4 5 6 7 8 9 10

> *"It may demand courage and self-discipline, but by freely acknowledging who we are, we can make positive changes about who we are becoming."*
>
> — Author unknown

I hope you are beginning to understand how holistic balance within these six components can enhance your life and work to decrease stress.

THE BALANCE WHEEL OF HEALTH AND WELL-BEING EXERCISE

The balance wheel of health and well-being exercise provides a visual representation of your level of satisfaction with your life. To

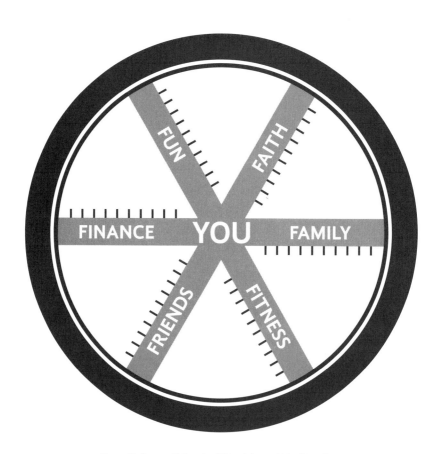

Your Balance Wheel of Health and Well-Being

complete this exercise, place an *X* on the spot best representing your present level of satisfaction with the specific spoke of the wheel. Use a scale of one to ten. The base of each spoke represents a low level of satisfaction, whereas the outer end represents a high level of satisfaction. Remember, there is no right or wrong.

After you have marked each component, connect the *X*'s on each spoke. Look at the wheel you created and ask yourself the following:

- Can my wheel roll smoothly?
- Am I completely deflated and riding on the rim?
- What components need to be reinflated?

How did you do? When I first completed the balance wheel exercise, my wheel was not round. Some who have completed the balance wheel exercise found they were riding on the rim. After viewing your balance wheel, can you understand what I mean when I say, "Flat wheels won't roll"?

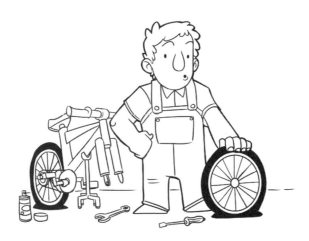

Flat Wheels Won't Roll

I encourage you to complete the exercises again after completing this book, in a year and then perhaps every year thereafter. Take time to look honestly at yourself and how you are living as you develop greater self-awareness, then implement simple strategies to improve yourself so you come to experience greater health, balance and abundance.

What's in It for Me?

As stated, the exercises are intended to create **A**wareness. When you begin to **A**ccept this new awareness, you will know and understand why changes may need to be made. If you want a satisfying life with good health, the exercises give you a place to start—a place from where you can begin to take **A**ction to move your life forward in a better and perhaps different direction. **A**wareness, **A**cceptance and **A**ction, known as the **Three A's**, are processes of change that require investments of time, effort and perseverance to obtain positive returns.

In the world of finance, **R**eturn **O**n **I**nvestment, or **ROI**, is a measure of the money earned on financial investments. Your **R**eturn **O**n **L**ife, or **ROL**, are the benefits received from the investments you make in your life. Your **ROL** is directly related to the **Three A's** you adopt and the habits you enforce daily, monthly and yearly. These investments made consistently over time affect your health and well-being. They will affect the returns you receive for living your life.

I realize it is difficult to make changes in the way we live and do things. To motivate myself, I ask, "What's in it for me?" When it comes to my life and health, I respond, "If I do not make better choices beginning now, in twenty or thirty years I may be dealing with a health and/or life condition that I had an eighty percent chance of preventing." My balance wheel may be partly deflated now, but with ongoing neglect, it will become a flat tire.

A Better **C**hoice for living life is to make wiser and more healthful choices now. When we make better choices to build strong and loving **F**amily and **F**riend relationships, when we engage in more healthful **F**itness and **F**inancial strategies and when we improve the **F**aith we have in ourselves and others, we receive an improved **R**eturn **O**n **L**ife. Our investments allow us to have more **F**un as our balance wheels roll smoothly.

You Have Choices

At the end of your day, do you *play back the tapes of your performance*? Do you reflect on the impact of your daily actions? How do the daily investments you make in your relationships, the food you eat and the thoughts you think affect the returns you receive? How do the sights you see, the sounds you hear and the words you read or speak affect how well your balance wheel of health and well-being rolls along?

> *"At the end of each day you should play back the tapes of your performance. The results should either applaud you or prod you."*
> — Jim Rohn (1930–2009), American entrepreneur, author and motivational speaker

Making good choices in a fast-paced world is not easy. Sometimes there are too many options to choose from. Sometimes we don't have enough information to base our decisions on, we don't like the choices available to us or our choices have simply become routines or bad habits. Stopping to thoroughly consider the future returns on the choices we make today may lead us to choose differently.

Picture yourself getting up in the morning: You may stretch, exercise and shower. You brush your teeth, dress and eat a nutritious breakfast. You may meditate or pray, take the dog for a walk and prepare food for your children. You may have housework to complete or give support and care to an aging parent.

As you head to work or appointments or run errands, there are traffic and weather conditions to deal with. Places of employment, healthcare centers and businesses all have people who are dealing with the particulars of their lives. You make choices about how you relate to them.

The day goes on—conversations, laughter and confrontations. You move from here to there, rushing to fit everything in before you go to the gym, go home to prepare another meal or take the car for service. You may attend night school, mow the lawn or take children to music lessons. You may help a family member, tend to pets or take out the garbage. You may meet friends or work on a special project. There are many actions and interactions to engage in every day. Each brings choices and consequences. Add to your day different crises—a cold, car problems or a family member's illness; problems with special projects, work concerns or even a major turn in the weather.

As you go about each new day, do you question why you are doing what you are doing? Why are you responding in a particular way? Do you ask, "How can I do this better?" or "Can I make **A B**etter **C**hoice?"

At the end of your day, do you play back the tapes of your performance?

If you do not stop to question your choices, you may not realize how your "normal" may be the unhealthful choices that will lead you to ride on the rim of life years later. At that point, all you may have the ability to do is stop your health and life issues from worsening. Simple healthful choices made continually today promote wellness while helping to prevent negative returns and illness tomorrow.

> *"A journey may be long or short, but it must start at the very spot one finds oneself."*
> — Jim Stovall, American author and speaker

What happens when you are ill? I know that when I'm ill, it impacts my life. It slows me down. It affects what I need and want to do, impacting the people I love, care for and work for. It affects my finances. I am unable to enjoy my family, keep my home in order or go out with friends. When I'm ill, I need to take time off work, and since I do not have sick benefits, my income decreases, impacting the funds available to buy groceries, pay bills and save for the future. I'm unable to enjoy life! Can you afford to be ill?

Knowing and being aware of yourself, your body and your thoughts may help you prevent future problems. Be aware and learn to recognize early warnings that can indicate there is something not right with you and your body. Make **A B**etter **C**hoice, knowing that *an ounce of prevention is worth a pound of cure.* There are better choices to be made every day that enable a healthier, balanced and more abundant life for you and your loved ones, now and into the future. When you and I make small, positive changes in how we manage life, future outcomes begin to change. Our **R**eturn **O**n **L**ife improves.

Changing your diet to include healthful, nutrient-rich foods noticeably improves your health in a few weeks. Beginning an exercise routine adds new vitality almost immediately. Reading positive, inspirational literature brings awareness and a new level of confidence. Responding lovingly to yourself and those around you improves relationships. The positive choices you practice regularly and consistently produce results to inspire more positive choices.

> *"If you do what you've always done, you'll get what you always got."*
>
> — Mark Twain (1835–1910), American author and humorist

Short-term actions multiplied by time equal long-term results. Consider the following:

- Who maintains a healthy weight, the one who speaks of all the benefits of exercise or the one who walks daily?

- Who retires early, the one who dreams of a house on the beach or the one who invests $200 a month?

- Who has the best marital relationship, the one who knows quality time improves relationships or the one who actually sits down and talks with their partner every night?

- Who writes a book, the one who dreams of becoming an author or the one who gets up early and writes for an hour a day?

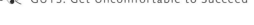

- Who has the most fun, the one who dreams about laughing and spending time with friends or the one who picks up the phone, goes out and works at making it happen?

"The best inspiration is not to outdo others, but to outdo ourselves."

— Author unknown

Remember, as a magnificent masterpiece, you can accomplish many great and wonderful things. You can reach your goals and potential as you become the best you can be.

The following chapters address our needs through the **Six F's**. They address how stress within each area impacts your health and well-being as your biography may well become your biology.

You may choose to read them in the order presented, or you may choose to read them in the order that interests you, as each chapter can stand on its own. However, please remember that balance between the **Six F's** will help you create a healthy, holistic life. Within each chapter, I hope you find a **TIP To Improve your Performance or A Better Choice to improve your Return On Life**.

I encourage you to think outside the box, keep an open mind and **Keep It Super Simple**. Be willing to regularly make small changes. Begin your journey at the very spot you find yourself.

A friend said to me, "I wasn't born this way. I learned to be this way." Learn to live life with the aid of basic life principles and practices that have stood the test of time. And remember that whatever is happening in your life, whatever challenges and difficulties you have, you can find a better way to respond to them by saying …

Let It Begin with Me!

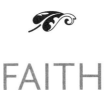

Chapter 3

FAITH

Faith as Part of Your Health- and Life-Care Systems

Some may be offended by my belief that faith is a vital component of our health and well-being because people often associate faith with religious practice. But for me, faith is not about structured religion. It is about belief. In the context of the Let It Begin with Me principle, it's the positive beliefs you have in yourself, in others, in life processes and in a higher spirit that are important.

Faith is seldom considered in discussions concerning health promotion. It is not part of many conversations and programs about disease prevention. But faith and belief are important and perhaps even essential components of our health- and life-care systems. Faith impacts our lives in many ways. It influences how we care for ourselves. Faith gives

> *"The only thing that stands between a man and what he wants from life is often merely the will to try it and the faith to believe that it is possible."*
>
> — Richard M. DeVos, American businessman and politician

people peace of mind. It brings contentment, satisfaction and calmness to our lives. Faith eases our acceptance of the uncertainties of life.

I believe we need faith in ourselves, others, life processes and a higher spirit to keep us grounded, stable and flexible in life. I believe faith helps us live healthier, balanced and more abundant lives.

Faith is a firm belief in an idea or outcome for which there is no irrefutable proof. It tends to arise from our experiences rather than from tangible evidence. Faith has not been proven scientifically, nor is it something we can see. It comes from our beliefs. It's about trust.

> **"Faith is to believe what we do not see."**
>
> — Augustine (354–430), Latin theologian and philosopher

Faith introduces us to *spirituality* and a higher spirit. But the view that spirituality is a prime element of our lives and a *spirit* protects us—watches over us—is often not accepted in a world searching for explanations and proof. However, studies indicate that people who have a spiritual component to their lives exhibit fewer self-destructive behaviors. Suicide, alcoholism and drug abuse, along with the various impacts of stress, are seen less often in spiritually minded people. Those who are spiritually minded have been known to experience a higher satisfaction with life, handle disease with greater ease and be healthier.

Having faith reduces depression, improves blood pressure and boosts the immune system. Faith promotes good health and fights disease by offering social supports and improving coping skills. In his book *God, Faith, and Health: Exploring the Spirituality-Healing Connection*, Jeff Levin, PhD, highlights different studies pointing out how faith or spiritually based practices help us live healthier lives.

- Johns Hopkins University researchers learned that monthly religious attendance more than halved the risk of death due to heart disease, emphysema, cirrhosis of the liver, suicide and some cancers.

- Patients in coronary care who were prayed for by strangers fared better than patients who didn't receive prayer.

- Mexican Americans who were church attendees reported higher levels of well-being and experienced less disability, fewer days in bed and fewer physical symptoms than non-churchgoers.

What we believe affects all areas of our lives and shapes every decision we make. One of the purposes behind the "I" statement and balance wheel exercises is to encourage you to take time to think about your beliefs, to ask how they were formed and how they affect your life and health. Our beliefs are the foundation on which we base our opinions and make our decisions and choices. They are like a mental filter through which all external information passes.

If there is contradiction between our beliefs and the way we live our lives, it creates uneasiness and dissatisfaction that affects our emotional and, ultimately, our physical well-being. This creates stress and keeps our bodies spinning too fast. Also, when our beliefs are not motivating, we can make unhealthful choices that may result in poor self-esteem and eventually lead to depression.

Douglas M. Lawson, PhD, says *the source of our personal power is our beliefs.* He emphasizes that what we believe to be true and how we feel about ourselves determines what we think we can do. He says, "Our belief system is, to a large extent, a collection of convictions we have about ourselves." When we think we are too weak, small or powerless to accomplish anything significant, we limit our experiences and outcomes in life.

> *"We cannot exercise our faith beyond what we believe to be possible."*
>
> — John G. Lake (1870–1935), Canadian missionary and faith healer

As we live our lives, challenges and struggles arise. We can become confused or lost in regards to what to do. During these times, faith will keep us moving forward. Faith in ourselves, others, life processes and a higher spirit guides us to make wise choices and have peace of mind. A strong faith prevents us from quitting and losing direction.

It may not always keep us from difficulty or trouble, but it helps us deal with those challenges more effectively. A healthful level of faith moves us forward and keeps our balance wheels inflated.

> *"Faith is not belief without proof, but trust without reservations."*
>
> — David Elton Trueblood (1900–1994), American Quaker, author and theologian

We all have some measure of faith. We have faith that a chair will hold us up when we sit in it. We have faith that when we put the key in the ignition of our car, it will start. We have faith our food will cook when we turn on the stove.

Few of us take time to think about the beliefs we accept to be true. Few take time to question if what we believe and trust in is actually healthful and good for us. Many of us inherit our beliefs and convictions from our parents, simply absorbing them without investigating or asking why. The beliefs of our parents and the people around us, or the messages the media give us, may not be right or even healthful for us, but we often accept them without stopping to question their validity. Some of us formulate unhealthful beliefs out of rebellion against the belief of others.

> *"Your belief determines your action and your action determines your results, but first you have to believe."*
>
> — Mark Victor Hansen, American speaker, trainer and author

What do you believe about yourself, others, life processes and a higher spirit? What are your beliefs on how life works? What do you believe when things don't work out the way you had hoped, when those around you aren't as supportive or understanding as you need them to be or when bad things happen to you or those you love? Do you believe everything will work out for the good, or do you believe the results will be negative?

When your belief system is put to the test, do you have the faith to persevere? Can you hold onto your faith in spite of difficulty, believing in new possibilities and finding comfort despite the unknowns? Do you believe events will work themselves out for the benefit of all concerned?

> *"Faith is the refusal to panic."*
>
> — David Martyn Lloyd-Jones (1899–1991), Welsh Protestant minister and medical doctor

FEAR

Many of our beliefs are based in fear, stopping us from believing in positive outcomes. Fear is an unpleasant, often strong emotion caused by the anticipation or awareness of danger or harm. Fear holds us back, limiting the way we respond to life and its challenges. Our beliefs concerning our possibilities, or their lack, control what we accomplish in life. When faced with difficulty, one person will say, "Let's work to find a solution," whereas many others will say, "It's impossible." Many of us walk away from doing more because we're told we are not capable and we believe it to be true.

> *"The only thing that separates any one of us from excellence is fear, and the opposite of fear is faith."*
>
> — Michael J. Fox, Canadian actor, author, producer and activist for Parkinson's disease

Fear affects our Faith. It prevents us from trusting and believing our challenges will turn out well. Fear affects how we relate to our Families and Friends, how we handle our Fitness and Finances and how we have Fun. Anytime we allow fear to get a grip on us, we become immobile instead of active. Fear freezes us in place, preventing progress and keeping us from stepping forward.

Fear is not simply an emotion or feeling. Fear affects us physically. In *Who Switched Off My Brain? Controlling Toxic Thoughts and Emotions*, Dr. Caroline Leaf reports that fear "triggers more than 1,400 known physical and chemical responses, activates more than 30 different hormones and neurotransmitters and is at the root of all stress." When fear causes a stress reaction in the body, it actually marinates the body in toxic chemicals, threatening our physical well-being. Fear, in its more advanced stages, can lead us to do irrational things. It can even lead to mental and emotional problems.

Our list of fears can be endless. We may fear pain, difficulty or sacrifice. We may fear losing friends, being alone or that no one will understand us. Fear can destroy our lives. As Dr. Leaf says, "Fear always tells you what you are not, what you do not have and what you cannot do, and what you never will be."

When we have fearful thoughts and feelings, they distract us and prevent us from enjoying life. Some people are so afraid of life they forget to live.

Don't let fear control you or prevent you from having a full and productive life. *Feel the fear and do it anyway*. When you make the choice to do it afraid, you move your life in a positive direction.

> **"We spend precious hours fearing the inevitable. It would be wise to use that time adoring our families, cherishing our friends and living our lives."**
>
> — Maya Angelou, American author and poet

The word *fear* means "to take flight or to run away from." When we are fearful we cower, shrink back and withdraw. Instead of having faith in ourselves, fear strips us of our self-confidence. Because of feelings of fear, many of us never reach our potential. It is better for our health and lives to fight fear with faith. As someone once said to me, "Fear knocked on my door. When faith answered, no one was there."

FEAR is an acronym for **F**alse **E**vidence **A**ppearing **R**eal. Is what you fear really real? Is your fear causing negative and unhealthful thoughts? Is fear leading you to **F**orget **E**verything **A**nd **R**un? What percentage of your fears actually happen?

Are you forgetting all the positive aspects about yourself, your capabilities and your world and running away because of fear? Or are you reminding yourself of all the good around you as a way to help guide your decisions, engage you in positive thinking and thrive?

When you become fearful, ask yourself, "Is what I fear really something that will hurt me and cause me pain, or is it only my thoughts telling me so?" Building your faith in yourself, others, life processes and a higher spirit can assist you in dealing with and alleviating your fears. Consider how many others have overcome fears and succeeded. Focus on successful outcomes as you either overcome your fear or do it despite your fear.

I went treetop trekking with my husband. Initially, it looked exciting, fun and safe. After climbing the first tree, fear of falling, fear of injury and fear of embarrassment set in. I was attached to a safety harness and we had a guide with us, and yet I was being controlled by **F**alse **E**vidence that **A**ppeared **R**eal to me. I wanted to **F**orget **E**verything I knew **A**nd **R**un.

> *"Fear is a condenser; love, an expander. This means that fear can create a world as small as a thimble, while love is able to open us to the fullness of living."*
>
> — Harold Klemp, American spiritual leader

Directly in front of me were two seventy-two-year-old women safely managing the treetop cables. That encouraged me. I continued moving along the cables, strengthened my confidence and completed the trekking experience. I continued to be fearful at times, but I persevered, did not give up and was successful in my endeavor.

Fear can stop us before we begin. We may believe we are less talented or capable than others. We may believe others are superior to us or believe we aren't smart enough, good enough or strong enough.

When we let fear take hold of us, we fall into the trap of settling for less in life. Fear of failure, of not being accepted or of making a mistake stops us from trying. Fear of looking foolish or unwise and fear of success are fears some of us face.

We each believe what we think to be true. Fears are self-limiting beliefs leading us to think we are deficient in some way. Self-limiting beliefs act as brakes on our potential. They stop us in our tracks, preventing us from taking the steps necessary to reach our goals. Remember, we're magnificent masterpieces, capable of much more than we often believe.

To become aware of your beliefs, learn to be observers of what you think, hear and say. Some of your thoughts and the comments you hear and say, no matter how well intended, can keep you from trying new experiences and living your life to the fullest.

> *"Don't be afraid to go out on a limb. That's where the fruit is."*
>
> — H. Jackson Brown Jr., American author

Many fears are fallacies we allow to control, accuse and condemn. Yes, there are some restrictions to what we can accomplish, but most of our fears can be exposed as **LIES**, or Limiting Ideas that Eliminate Success. They block us as soon as we hit an obstacle or a bump in the road.

To prevent these **LIES** from affecting you, consider making a **LIAR** out of them by saying, "Let's Inspire Another Response." Instead of saying, "I can't learn something new" or "I'm not smart enough," inspire another response by saying, "I can learn to do new things. I can do this!"

Instead of saying, "I'll never be able to get through the trials I am facing," inspire another response by saying, "I will focus only on what needs to be accomplished today. In doing so, I know I will be able to handle the challenges I am facing."

Instead of saying, "He/she's not the man/woman I married. I don't love him/her anymore so I'm going to divorce him/her," inspire another response by saying, "I will focus on all his/her good qualities and let him/her know how wonderful he/she is. I know marriage is not always easy. I will put more effort into our relationship and create a marriage that survives the test of time."

Fear has been a big obstacle in my life. Fear has led me to hide, procrastinate and belittle myself. Fear of looking foolish has stopped me from trying a new activity. Fear of hurting someone's feelings has stopped me from speaking up when my feelings were hurt or injustices have occurred. Fear of losing or damaging a relationship has led me to respond in ways where I lose my self-respect. My fears and accompanying responses never bring the results I desire. In fact, I find fear creates more fear, diminishing my joy and opportunity to lead a fulfilling life.

Fear is not a sign of weakness or cowardice, but an emotion we must respond to. It requires a decision and an action. Learning ways to challenge our fears will inspire us to respond differently. Changing our thoughts and our actions helps diminish our fears.

> *"Courage is fear that has said its prayers."*
> — Dorothy Bernard (1890–1955), American actress

When I recognize I'm responding to fear, I'll acknowledge it, consider my options and tell myself, "I can overcome this." I remember how I've overcome a fear and obstacle in the past. I believe that when I've overcome before, I can overcome again. Then I take positive action steps to move myself forward.

Education helps decrease our enslavement to fear. It opens the doors to new opportunities and choices while increasing our faith and confidence in ourselves.

The acronym **KASH**, explained in Denis Waitley's book *Safari to the Soul*, provides a way to inspire another response to fear. When we improve our **K**nowledge, **A**ttitude, **S**kills and **H**abits, we enhance our lives.

> *"I believe that anyone can conquer fear by doing the things they fear to do, provided they keep doing them until they get a record of successful experiences behind them."*
> — Eleanor Roosevelt (1884–1962), First Lady of the United States from 1933 to 1945

- **K**nowledge: Increasing our knowledge and understanding of a particular subject, activity or person helps combat fear while building greater confidence in ourselves.

- **A**ttitude: Positive attitudes move us forward, whereas negative attitudes stop us and hold us back.

- **S**kills: New skills are learned by observing, imitating and doing, leading to improved confidence and decreased fear. Remember, *there never was a winner who was not first a beginner*.

- **H**abits: Habits are unconscious patterns of behavior. A habit of negative thinking leads to fear. Changing habits takes time, but keep in mind, *by the inch, success is a cinch; by the yard, it's hard*.

Faith in Self: The Relationship You Have with Yourself

Living life well requires having faith in ourselves. Faith in ourselves requires us to love the person we are. We may need to learn how to love ourselves. But we can learn to love ourselves only when we are willing to search out who we truly are. Then we will develop a healthy self-image, which is foundational to our success and happiness.

Remember, you are a magnificent masterpiece; your mere existence is a miracle. Every day when you wake up, when your heart beats and when you breathe, you are accomplishing something phenomenal, outstanding and wonderful. Acknowledging how exquisitely you are made and the great potential you hold within you builds confidence and belief in yourself. It strengthens your self-image and builds your faith.

> *"Love yourself first and everything falls into line."*
> — Lucille Ball (1911–1989), American actress

Positive belief and faith in ourselves counteract the negative self-talk many frequently engage in. When we focus on the negative, we rob ourselves of our future success. Positive belief and faith in ourselves provides the fuel, energy and persistence we need to act, make better choices and move in a positive direction.

I Believe

I believe every person has within themselves
inexhaustible reserves of potential they have
never even come close to realizing.

I believe each person has far more
intelligence than they have ever used.

I believe each person is more creative
than he or she has ever imagined.

I believe the greatest achievements
of your life lie ahead of you.

I believe the happiest moments
of your life are yet to come.

I believe the greatest successes you will ever attain
are still waiting for you on the road ahead.

And, I believe through learning and
application of what you learn, you can solve any
problem, overcome any obstacle and achieve
any goal that you can set for yourself.

— Brian Tracy, Canadian author and motivational speaker

We all have a need to be loved and desire love, but if we don't love ourselves and show love for ourselves, it is difficult to give true love to others. We can't give away something we don't have. When we love ourselves, we take care of our own needs in a healthful way, and we are able to love others in healthful ways.

Love is a decision and an action. It is a decision we make on how we will act toward ourselves and others.

When your beliefs about yourself are rooted in feelings of shame, guilt, inferiority, rejection or numerous other negative feelings, your relationship with yourself and others suffers. This is not love. We each need to learn to like, love and accept ourselves for the person we are; in doing so we increase our joy in life. But we need to do this in a balanced way, not in a selfish or self-centered way. Love yourself, but don't be *in love* with yourself; enable your love to flow through you to others.

Loving yourself is **A B**etter **C**hoice for your health and life**.** To sum up, when you take action to **LOVE** yourself, you

- **L**isten and **L**earn what your needs are,

- **O**verlook your faults,

- **V**alidate and **V**alue how amazing and worthy you are, and then put

- **E**ffort and **E**nergy into caring for yourself.

> *"There is no fear in love. But perfect love drives out fear, because fear has to do with punishment."*
>
> — 1 John 4:18

Here are some other **TIP**s to build faith and love in yourself:

- Think positively about yourself; the way you think about yourself reveals how you feel about yourself and often makes it a reality.

- Say good things about yourself; be your own best friend.

- Don't compare yourself with other people—everyone in the world is unique; don't compete with who you think others are—be yourself.

- Focus on your potential instead of your limitations; we all have individual gifts—work on yours.

- Find something you like and would like to do well, and then do it over and over; *practice makes perfect.*

- Have the courage to be different and deal with the criticism; you won't like yourself when you go against your own convictions.

- Don't let the way another person treats you determine or steal away your self-worth; don't be controlled by what others say, do and think.

- Keep your flaws in perspective; no one is perfect.

- Love how your body works more than how it looks; take good care of your body by

  - eating healthful foods,

  - exercising regularly,

  - getting a good night's sleep,

  - visiting your doctor and dentist for regular checkups,

  - building positive relationships, and

  - laughing and having fun.

Faith in Others: The Relationship You Have with the People in Your Life

We all need people in our lives. We need to feel a sense of community and belonging to a group or a family of others. Because of this, it's easy to become too involved in other people's lives. It feels good when we help others and feel needed. The challenge is to set reasonable and effective boundaries and to know the difference between our responsibilities and someone else's.

Research at the University of Wales Lampeter showed that helping others has health benefits that include increased longevity, a sense of self, stress control and pain reduction. The studies showed that the body

> *"People are different from each other ... no amount of getting after them is going to change them. Nor is there any reason to change them, because their differences are probably good."*
>
> — David Keirsey, American psychologist and author

releases endorphins, creating what some call the "helper's high."[1] However, when we become too involved in other people's lives, we do them a disservice. We prevent them from learning about themselves, their capabilities and their potential. We prevent them from growing and excelling.

Everyone has their own life to live and can do so in whatever way they choose. Each person has their own balance wheel to care for and move forward. It is neither our right nor our responsibility to do it for them. When we do too much for others, we deny them the opportunity to learn and grow. As Mark Twain said, "A man who carries a cat by the tail learns something he can learn in no other way."

There are times when other people need help, but, ultimately, they are responsible for maintaining, balancing and living their own lives. Demonstrating faith in another's ability to manage themselves begins with boundary lines that permit them to take responsibility and work out the consequences of their actions.

> **"We can help one another to find the meaning of life ... But in the last analysis, the individual person is responsible for living his own life and for 'finding himself.'"**
>
> — Thomas Merton (1915–1968), American author, activist and monk

When we control other people's lives, it takes our energy away. If you carry a backpack with your belongings, and then add the belongings of others, the load becomes heavy. The same is true when you carry other people's responsibilities. Becoming too involved with other people's lives makes you weary and lose focus in your life. We each need to trust and have faith in how others make decisions for themselves.

Steven Covey makes this point in his book *The Speed of Trust: The One Thing That Changes Everything*. He says we waste

---

1. Rachel Casiday, Eileen Kinsman, Clare Fisher, and Clare Bambra, "Volunteering and Health: What Impact Does It Really Have?" *Volunteering England* (July 2008), www.volunteering.org.uk/NR/rdonlyres/AB46F9EC-CADB-4ABB-AEFE-8A850F09AE32/0/FullReportLampeter2ndJuly2008.pdf.

much less of our life's energy when we manage our relationships from the perspective of trust. Occasionally, we will get hurt, but if we are resilient in our sense and love of self, we will easily recover. Life's a better place when we assume others are good and can be trusted.

The acronym **DETACH** stands for **D**on't **E**ven **T**hink **A**bout **C**hanging **H**im/**H**er. It reinforces the fact that people don't change unless they want to, and doing too much for them or offering unsolicited advice is futile.

Our lives are closely intertwined with those whom we love and care for. We may question whether letting go of someone else's balance wheel is even possible, but staying out of the affairs of others is more healthful for all concerned. It creates greater peace of mind. Living your life and letting others live their own is **A B**etter

> *"I honor and salute the magnificence in you. I honor the place in your heart where lives your courage, honor, love, hope and dreams. I honor the place in you where, if you are at that place in you and I am at that place in me, there is only one of us."*
>
> — Tibetan greeting

Choice for your health and well-being, so I suggest you **MYOB**, **M**ind **Y**our **O**wn **B**usiness. Ask yourself, "What is my responsibility in this matter?" and "What is their responsibility?" It will guide you in knowing where to set the boundary lines of involvement. *Instead of minding other people's business, create some business of your own to mind.*

Faith in Life Processes: Patience

Our society tends to demand instant gratification: instant coffee, instant breakfast, instant money. We want things fast and we want them now, decreasing our ability to be patient. Margaret Thatcher, past prime minister of England, said, "You may have to fight a battle more than once to win it!" Yet, when we try something and fail to see results quickly or confront obstacles, many of us give up.

Faith in the processes of life is about patience. It is about having faith in time. Faith in the time it takes to get things done. In the time it takes to change, grow and heal, along with the time it takes to overcome life's trials.

> *"Whoever is out of patience is out of possession of his soul."*
> — Jonathan Swift (1667–1745), Anglo-Irish satirist, essayist, poet and cleric

When you cut yourself or have surgery, it takes time for the incision to heal. The time for this process to be complete depends on the length and depth of the incision, whether infection sets in and the health of your body. After a heart attack, your heart needs time to heal and become stronger before you can go back to work and resume activities. Your body heals itself through a predefined process of healing. You can't speed up the time it takes. You need to wait.

Events and life take time to unfold and progress. Learning to trust and have confidence in the time it takes comes as we banish feelings of impatience, discouragement and impossibility. This, in turn, happens through perseverance, determination and not giving in.

We each need to be patient with ourselves, other people and time, since life does not happen in *our* time; it happens in *due* time. Patience is not just the ability to wait; it is the ability to keep a good attitude while waiting.

I am not always very patient. I can become agitated, frustrated and discouraged with the time it takes me to accomplish or learn something new, or the time it takes for others to do the same. When I'm working on a project, I often think I can complete it in less time than needed, but I've learned that when I lose patience and begin to force outcomes, the results are not what I had hoped for, and I feel regretful. When I want to give up entirely, my husband will say, "Betty, you don't need to throw out the baby with the bathwater!" Through the process of learning new behaviors, and with the aid of time, I am becoming better at waiting, and waiting with a good attitude.

Life and learning is a process. Children provide us with a great example of this. When children begin to walk, they grab hold of something and pull themselves up before they take a step. Inevitably they fall, but they get up again. The process of learning to walk takes time. We have faith in the process and the time it takes for children to learn to walk, so we encourage them. We know they will stumble and fall, but they will eventually walk. Waiting for them to do so is part of the process.

When we decide to become physically fit and lose weight, we begin a diet and exercise routine—eating more fruits and vegetables, taking a daily walk, working to get our heart rates up and adding weights. Stepping on the scale after a week, we may see only a slight change in weight. This may cause us to become discouraged, but we must remind ourselves it takes time to lose weight, strengthen our bodies and become physically fit. It takes consistent daily actions, discipline and commitment. It takes patience and understanding of processes to keep doing what needs to be done to attain desired results.

With patience, time can be our friend and work with us; without it, time can become our enemy and work against us. When we persist and do our part, time takes care of the rest. Understanding and respecting the power of time builds faith in the processes of life.

> *"And let us not lose heart and grow weary and faint in acting nobly and doing right, for in due time and at the appointed season we shall reap, if we do not loosen and relax our courage and faint."*
> — Galatians 6:9

Consider the analogy of a stonecutter splitting a rock. He may strike the rock ninety-nine times with no results, yet when he strikes one more blow, it splits in two. It's not the last strike that splits the rock, it was the ninety-nine plus one blows.

A bamboo tree is an amazing sight to see, soaring over 100 feet straight up. What's even more amazing about a bamboo tree is how it grows. Beginning with a bamboo stalk about eighteen inches long, a three-foot hole is dug and the stalk is buried completely in the ground. For the next five years, the stalk is watered every day. If one day is missed, the tree may never appear. But when meticulous care is taken for those five years, on the 1,825th day, the ground breaks open and the tree appears.

> *"Rome was not built in a day."*
>
> — Sixteenth-century proverb

What happens next is the phenomenon of the bamboo tree. The tree will soar to over ninety feet in a matter of six weeks. It grows at a rate of three feet every twenty-four hours. You can practically sit back and watch it grow. Some people say it takes six weeks for a bamboo tree to grow, whereas others say it takes five years and six weeks. The general principle behind the story of the bamboo tree is that one needs a lot of patience, not just action, to make things happen.

Faith in a Higher Spirit

A jogger nears the end of his run. To the left are sand dunes blocking his view of the beach beyond. If he were to cross the dunes, it would require extra effort after a long, tiring workout, but his route would be easier by remaining on the flat road veering away from the water. The jogger hesitates as an inner nudge urges him toward the dunes. He chooses to respond to it, and when the beach appears, he sees a spectacular sunset hovering above the crashing waves. Humility overwhelms him as he realizes, in his moment of hesitation, he had listened to a power greater than himself, one that could see around blind corners.

Having faith in a higher spirit or a power greater than ourselves lets us know we are not alone. It enables us to focus on a force we can call and rely on for understanding, strength and guidance. Whether we call this entity a higher power, God, Buddha, Creator, Allah, Jesus Christ, the universe or another name, studies show that having faith and belief in something greater than ourselves is good for our health.

However you choose to name it, for the purpose of this book, I identify this entity as higher spirit or God.

Eighty-five percent of the world's population believes there is a God. But of this number, how many understand the value of faith in a higher spirit in relation to creating a healthy, balanced and abundant life?

The work of Dr. Jeff Levin embraces the idea of the connection between faith in a higher spirit and health. Without promoting a particular spiritual point of view, his research studies explore the connection between health and various spiritual beliefs and practices. It shows that people who have faith in a God, or who engage in spiritual practices such as prayer or meditation, attending religious services or using healing rituals as a reflection of their faith, experience better health.

Cars have shock absorbers to soften the blow of unexpected potholes. Faith in a higher spirit can act as a shock absorber, giving comfort and softening the many potholes we encounter in life. Some may feel left alone to handle their challenges and disappointments, but when we have faith in a higher spirit, we are never alone. This higher spirit is always there to offer us unconditional love and to protect, direct and correct our actions.

When we need to reason everything out, we may have difficulty coming to a position of faith. But when we stop needing reasons to explain all of the mysteries of our world, we begin to find our faith. When we begin to rely on something other than ourselves, our possibilities are expanded by this unseen presence.

"There is guidance for each of us, and by lowly listening, we shall hear the right word. Certainly there is a right for you that needs no choice on your part. Place yourself in the middle of the stream of power and wisdom which flows into your life. Then, without effort, you are impelled to truth and to perfect contentment."

— Ralph Waldo Emerson (1803–1882), American essayist, lecturer and poet

"Every now and again take a good look at something not made with hands—a mountain, a star, the turn of a stream. There will come to you wisdom and patience and solace and, above all, the assurance that you are not alone in the world."

— Sidney Lovett (1890–1979), American clergyman and chaplain

Studies confirm that the belief in a higher spirit can have a profound effect on people's mental state, their ability to cope with illness, the speed at which they recover from a medical disorder, the strength of their immune systems and the hope and optimism they find as they practice their particular form of spirituality. One study involving older adults undergoing heart surgery found that those who were engaged in religious or spiritual practices were three times less likely to die within six months after surgery than those who weren't.[2]

Seventh-day Adventists are instructed by their church not to consume alcohol or pork or smoke tobacco. In a ten-year study, researchers found that Adventists lived longer than the national average and the chance of their dying from cancer or heart disease was much lower than the national average.[3]

The act of putting oneself in the presence of or conversing with a spiritual entity or praying has been used as a means of healing across most cultures throughout the ages. Today, many people believe that prayer or meditation is an important part of daily life. According to a survey of 1,000 American physicians, eighty-five percent believe religion or spiritual practices positively influence patients' health and recovery.[4]

---

2. Thomas E. Oxman, Daniel H. Freeman Jr., and Eric D. Manheimer, "Lack of Social Participation or Religious Strength and Comfort as Risk Factors for Death after Cardiac Surgery in the Elderly," *Psychosomatic Medicine* 5, no. 1 (1995): 5–15.

3. Terry L. Butler et al., "Cohort Profile: The Adventist Health Study-2 (AHS-2)," *International Journal of Epidemiology* 37, no. 2 (2008): 260–265.

4. Robert Shmerling, "Can Prayer Heal the Sick?" *Harvard Health Publications* (2009), http://health.msn.com/health-topics/articlepage.aspx?cp-documentid=100244053.

Researchers have also studied intercessory and distance prayer, which is asking God to intervene on behalf of another, either known or unknown to the person praying. When compared with those who were not prayed for, patients who were prayed for showed general improvements in the course of their illness, fewer complications and even fewer deaths.[5]

Programs with a strong spiritual component, such as various twelve-step programs, show that spirituality is effective in dealing with addictions. The regular practice of prayer and meditation is strongly associated with recovery and abstinence from addictive behaviors.

Each spiritual denomination has their sacred books to provide philosophies and insights about living life. Islam has the Koran; Hinduism has the Vedas, Mahabharata and Ramayana; Buddhism has the Sutras; Judaism has the Torah and the Old Testament; and Christianity has the Bible. These special books give their readers and followers guidance on how to live life well and how to develop strong, supportive and loving relationships with others. The acronym **BIBLE**, **B**asic **I**nstruction **B**efore **L**eaving **E**arth, illustrates the intent and value of these books.

A relationship with a higher spirit or God seems to add an extra dimension to our lives. It can revitalize, energize and give peace of mind. As this may be difficult to comprehend, an explanation from a colleague may help you understand. "God might be likened to the electricity that operates the lights and machinery of my life. It's not necessary to understand what electricity actually is for me to enjoy its use—all I need to do is turn on the switch!"

> *"Do your best and let God do the rest!"*
> — Ben Carson, American neurosurgeon

Another friend said, "Having faith and trusting in God helps me not obsess about outcomes to situations and not be bitterly disappointed when things don't turn out the way

5. Ibid.

I hoped they would. By turning things over to God and trusting Him, I let go of attachments and feel more at peace with myself, my life and my world."

I grew up believing in a God of punishment more than a God of love. That belief locked me into strong feelings of guilt, shame and low self-esteem for many years. Today I have come to believe in a God of love and possibilities. My God loves and accepts me unconditionally. He provides me with the guidance and wisdom I need to make choices that are good for me, my life and those I care for. He helps me accept and love myself and others for the people we are.

> *"The intellect has little to do on the road to discovery. There comes a leap in consciousness, call it intuition or what you will, and the solution comes to you and you don't know how or why."*
>
> — Albert Einstein (1879–1955), German theoretical physicist

My God gives me peace of mind, contentment and strength. He is a God of everyday use and is always available and loving. When life becomes busy and complicated, I'll pull away to connect with my God. This helps me find solutions that enable my life to flow smoother, stabilize and be balanced. When I ask my God for guidance and keep myself receptive for a loving response, the decisions I make guide me to overcome my challenges and difficulties.

Building a relationship with God, just as with any relationship, takes time. If you are interested in building a relationship with a higher spirit but do not know where to begin, a comfortable place to start may be to consider the well-known acronym **GOD**, **G**ood **O**rderly **D**irection. Asking and searching for **G**ood **O**rderly **D**irection can open the door to knowledge, wisdom and understanding that, in turn, guides you to make more healthful choices and take positive actions.

Another simple way to find and build a relationship with a higher spirit is by saying, "Good morning, God" every morning, even if you do not believe it. One morning when you say it, you may believe there is a God who hears you and loves you.

I believe a higher spirit or God is revealed to us in various ways—through our intuition, thoughts and feelings, and through literature, music and even people. We only need to be receptive by listening and hearing.

The love and guidance of God has added value to many people's lives. It is a treasure many find priceless as they receive support and direction for their daily lives. They remain calm and peaceful knowing their God has become like a loving parent or best friend who is there all the time, providing courage, strength and hope to enhance their daily activities and interactions.

As stated earlier, we need to have a positive self-image in order to thrive. On the other hand, it is equally important that we do not allow our **EGO**s to **E**ase **G**od **O**ut. Our egos may get us thinking of ourselves as separate from the world and may prevent us from developing a relationship with a higher spirit because we believe we can handle life on our own.

Thich Nhat Hanh, a Buddhist monk and philosopher, states, "Without a spiritual dimension, we will not have the capacity to confront suffering, to transform suffering and to offer anything to life. A person without a spiritual path is a person walking in darkness. With a spiritual path, we are no longer afraid or worried." When we **E**ase **G**od **O**ut of our lives, we may diminish our capacity to accept life for what it is and others for who they are. Incorporating a higher spirit into our lives takes us from indifference to compassion and from fear to love.

Consider setting your **GOALS** with the guidance of a higher spirit as a way to enhance your relationship with a spiritual entity and your effectiveness in achieving your potential. **G**od's **O**bjectives **A**lways **L**ead to **S**uccess. Time and time again, I have found the answers I receive by asking my God for help and direction lead to good outcomes. By listening for morally and ethically sound answers, I am led to choices and opportunities that give me peace of mind. When I have not taken the time to connect with my higher spirit and listen for answers, I stumble and falter. Going to my God before making my decisions helps me feel secure and leads to many successes.

Please note that direction from a higher spirit doesn't necessarily come in the form of easy solutions. Each of us must play a part in solving our own problems and handling our life challenges. We must also use sound judgment, intelligence, goodwill and the power of reason to make wise decisions. In doing so, we must not be resentful or fail to face our issues honestly. We need to be tolerant of the faults of others and not become emotional over our problems. When we are open, God provides the guidance and the strength for us to make decisions and take the loving actions needed to best suit our particular situation. I have come to know that when I do my part, my God will not take me where His love will not protect me. *Seeking God's presence and not God's presents leads to peace of mind.*

> *"I have held many things in my hands, and I have lost them all; but whatever I have placed in God's hands, that I still possess."*
>
> — Martin Luther (1483–1546), German priest and professor of theology

The following poem is a favorite of mine. It came my way over twenty years ago and reflects how I have seen my God work in my life through the years, through numerous trials and tribulations. It reflects how I see my relationship with Him today.

The Road of Life

At first, I saw God as my observer, my judge,
keeping track of the things I did wrong,
so as to know whether I merited heaven or hell when I die.
He was out there sort of like a president. I recognized

His picture when I saw it,
but I really didn't know Him.

But later on when I truly met God, it seemed as
though life were rather like a bike ride,
but it was a tandem bike, and I noticed that God
was in the back helping me pedal.

I don't know just when it was that
He suggested we change places,
but life has not been the same since.

When I had control, I knew the way,
it was rather boring, but predictable ...
It was the shortest distance between two points.

But when He took the lead, He knew
delightful long cuts, up mountains,
and through rocky places at breakneck speeds,
it was all I could do to hang on!
Even though it looked like madness, He said, "Pedal!"

I worried and was anxious and asked,
"Where are you taking me?"
He laughed and didn't answer, and
I started to learn to trust.

I forgot my boring life and entered
into the adventure.
And when I'd say, "I'm scared,"
He'd lean back and touch my hand.

He took me to people with gifts that I needed, gifts
of healing, acceptance and joy.
They gave me gifts to take on my journey, my Lord's
and mine. And we were off again.

He said, "Give the gifts away; they're extra baggage,
too much weight." So I did, to the people we met,
and I found that in giving I received,
and still our burden was light.

I did not trust Him, at first, in control of my life.
I thought He'd wreck it;
but He knows bike secrets, knows how to
make it bend to take sharp corners,
knows how to jump to clear high rocks, knows how
to fly to shorten scary passages.

And I am learning to shut up and
pedal in the strangest places,
and I'm beginning to enjoy the view
and the cool breeze on my face
with my delightful constant companion,
my Lord, my God.

And when I'm sure I just can't do anymore,
He just smiles and says … "Pedal."

— **Author unknown**

Faith Takes Action

Faith is not a matter of chance; it is a matter of choice. It is not passive. Faith expressed only in our thoughts and words is not faith. Faith needs to be accompanied by actions.

I can talk about faith in myself, others, life processes or a higher spirit, but unless I do something, unless I take action based on faith, no matter the circumstances or my feelings, I do not demonstrate faith.

In his audiobook *Achieving Real Balance,* Ben Kubassek says, "Belief is believing that an egg yolk will turn into a chicken. Faith is the action of putting that egg into an incubator and trusting it will hatch." He says belief is believing every seed contains a harvest, whereas faith is shown through planting the seed, maintaining it and preparing it for harvest. Action is the difference between belief and faith. Our beliefs control our thoughts, but faith is what leads us to act. He says, "Beliefs help us draw the map, but faith inspires us to start the journey."

Developing faith takes time. It builds as we use it, experience it and stay the course, whether we fully believe in what we are doing or not. When we act in faith we begin something and move toward its completion.

As I write this book, I show my faith by my actions. I have faith and I believe that by creating awareness about holistic, balanced living and providing **TIP**s on how to work toward achieving it, you will make choices to change your life in a healthful and positive way. I do not know this for certain, but I show my faith when I research, edit and continue to bring the writing of this book to completion. Even though I am not always confident I can do this, or do it well, I press on and keep *pedaling*!

As a first-time author and inexperienced writer, logic may tell me not to expect much or to stop the process, but I move forward as my inner voice urges me to continue. Through my actions, I show faith and push myself to overcome my doubts and fears. I continue to rise early and use vacation time and weekends to write. I have even risked committing myself full time to its completion. This is how I act in faith.

> *"Action eradicates fear. No matter what you fear, positive, self-affirming action can diminish or completely cancel that which you are fearful of."*
> — Mark Victor Hansen, American speaker, trainer and author

> *"Whatever you can do or think you can do, begin it because boldness has magic, power and genius in it!"*
> — Henry David Thoreau (1817–1862), American author, poet and philosopher

I believe one of the best things I can do is to **PUSH** myself into action. I will simply **P**ray **U**ntil **S**omething **H**appens. I pray for the strength, wisdom and direction I need to complete this book and bring it to you. I pray for the right concepts, words and flow of ideas; I pray for the right research articles, acronyms and verses; and then I pray for the right strategies, connections and opportunities for the success of this manuscript. Then I take the necessary action steps as I follow through. I pray that you enjoy the read and the ideas and **TIP**s, and that you then take actions **T**o **I**mprove your **P**erformance in life and health.

Prayer is faith in action. Prayer is something we can do anywhere and anytime. We can pray out loud or silently. We can pray in a conversational fashion or through a set of memorized words. We can pray while walking, driving or in a business meeting. Our prayers can be long or just a few affirming words. We can pray while in a challenging confrontation, at a special event or in private. We can pray for guidance, peace of mind or help for ourselves and others. We can pray when we are angry, confused or upset, or when we are worried, lost or depressed. Calling out "help" works great for me. I know my God hears me, understands me and meets me wherever I am.

When we pray and receive answers or guidance, we must remain cognizant that healthful responses are those that demonstrate love for ourselves, others and this world. The **G**ood **O**rderly **D**irection we receive must be accompanied by actions that lead to healthy and loving results.

Embracing Health, Balance and Abundance through Your Faith

Faith in yourself, others, life processes and a higher spirit will enhance your life as it adds greater excitement, experiences and opportunities to living. As you show **LOVE** toward yourself, others and your **GOD**, your faith will aid you in addressing your fears while opening the door to new and wonderful opportunities. Whether it's how you view your self-image, show love unconditionally to others or make your choices and decisions, faith in these areas adds a new dimension to your life.

Building your faith may require times of personal discomfort as you take action steps in spite of your **FEAR**. Remember, it takes **GUTS** to inspire and implement another response. It takes **GUTS** to make a **LIAR** out of the **F**alse **E**vidence that **A**ppears **R**eal to you. It takes **GUTS** to stop yourself from **F**orgetting **E**verything **A**nd **R**unning away. In doing so, you may find the need to pray as you **PUSH** yourself into action while you build and strengthen your faith.

I encourage you to continue to journey through your life with the **G**ood **O**rderly **D**irection of a loving higher spirit as you build a better life for yourself, your family and those around you. I encourage you to persistently and faithfully say ...

Let It Begin with Me!

Chapter 4

FAMILY

What Is FAMILY?

From *Father Knows Best* to *Leave It to Beaver* to *The Brady Bunch* to *The Simpsons* to *Keeping Up with the Kardashians* to *Modern Family*, through time we have seen many different images of what families look like. They come in all shapes, sizes and structures, with many dynamics and many personalities. Some seem to run smoothly, others not so. But no matter what, we all desire a good family life with loving relationships, often based in one way or another on the family we grew up in.

Our initial experience with family is the one we're born into. In his book *The Ultimate Gift*, Jim Stovall writes, "Families give us our roots, our heritage, and our past. They also give us the springboard for our

> *"Lots of people are thrilled about the families they came from, others couldn't get away fast enough. Most people fall into that vast middle ground: great affection mixed with a few ideas for improvement. A couple of things they wish could have perhaps been done differently."*
>
> — Paul Reiser, American comedian, actor, author and musician

future." He says nothing is stronger than the family bond because it is "a bond of pure love that will withstand any pressure as long as love is kept in the forefront." However, often the "bond of pure love" is tested.

Some of us live our entire lives as part of the family we were born into. Others, because of divorce and remarriage, have new families added to their original families. Whereas others, through various circumstances, are left without family other than in name, generating a need to go out and create a family not related by blood, but by love.

Webster's describes *family* in a variety of ways as

- a group of people,

- a household unit of related people,

- a social group made up of parents and children,

- a group of persons living under one roof, and

- a group of persons that come from the same ancestor.

In my acronym dictionary, **FAMILY** stands for **F**ather **A**nd **M**other, **I L**ove **Y**ou. But the reality of life is that some parents don't always know how to show love in a nurturing and supportive way. Some don't know how to care for and support family members with acceptance, kindness, compassion and understanding. Perhaps as children they did not receive the acceptance, kindness, compassion and understanding they needed, or they received a distorted, unhealthful form of love, or they did not receive unconditional love. Whether loving or not, our families of origin play an important role in our lives.

Many families have become complicated and complex. They include parents and children as well as step-parents, step-children, step-grandparents, half brothers and sisters, ex-spouses and extended family members. They can be separated by long distances and unresolved issues. If it's not issues with divorce, it's parents who both work outside the home. If it's not child abuse, it's emotional neglect. If it's not alcoholism in parents, it's drug use by children. If it's not a lack of values in the older generation, it's lack of ambition in the younger generation. The list goes on, including that in some areas of North America nearly four out of ten children are raised in families without fathers, and one out of every four children before the age of sixteen lives with a step-parent.

Broken and dysfunctional environments are not easy places to live and grow up in. When we are in or have been part of these types of environments, we often bring a broken heart and pain with us into the adult world.

Whether we're raised in a nuclear family or a fragmented one, unresolved issues provoke unwholesome feelings within us. Feelings of anger and hurt and of being victimized, disappointed or betrayed may be carried with us long into our adult lives, and then they are passed on through future generations. If these feelings are unaddressed, they often resurface and can show up in stress-related illnesses such as heart conditions, cancer, respiratory problems, stomach and bowel problems, depression and anxiety.

A close family unit that lends help and emotional support has been found to offer protection against illness and disease. Researchers have found people who experience love and support tend to resist unhealthful behaviors and feel less stressed. In a clinical study of a close-knit Italian-American community, researchers found the death rate from heart attack was half the nation's average. Researchers concluded this strong social support network helped protect this population from heart disease.[1]

We all have a need and a desire to feel respected, supported and loved by our family members. If not resolved, problems within families may accumulate, creating baggage that gets stuffed into the family memory chest. Eventually, the trunk becomes so full it finally

1. Brenda Egolf et al., "The Roseto Effect: A 50-Year Comparison of Mortality Rates," *American Journal of Public Health* 82, no. 8 (1992): 1089–1092.

pops open, and the unresolved hurts, disappointments and other feelings resurface, creating tension, strife and even disease.

Many have heard the motto "You can choose your friends, but not your family." We are each born into a family not of our choosing. Learning how to love our family members and to communicate in ways in which we can maintain our individuality while still feeling welcome and appreciated goes a long way in building healthy families.

In this chapter I highlight some basic components of family relationships, including topics such as building and maintaining loving relationships, raising children, communicating effectively, addictions, abuse and forgiveness.

What Does LOVE Look Like?

Just shower the people you love with love

Show them the way that you feel

Things are gonna work out fine if you only will.

— James Taylor, American singer and songwriter

James Taylor, an American singer and songwriter, suggests we "shower the people we love with love." But what is love?

Webster's defines *love* as "to hold dear"; "affection based on admiration, benevolence, or common interests"; and "warm attachment."

Thomas Merton said, "The beginning of love is to let those we love be perfectly themselves, and not to twist them to fit our own image. Otherwise we love only the reflection of ourselves we find in them." He says loving others is accepting them for who they are.

Love is often associated with feelings, but love is shown through actions. It is a decision about how we will treat others. It's an act of our will, resulting in loving behavior, regardless of how we feel.

Just as the acronym **LOVE** was used to illustrate love of self, it can be used to create an image of what loving others looks like:

- **L**isten to and **L**earn what our loved ones value and need.

- **O**verlook flaws and faults in favor of seeing the good.

- **V**alidate and **V**alue by consistently approving with encouragement and praise.

- **E**ffort and **E**nergy are needed by spending time and showing our interest.

> *"Don't assume that money, shelter and creature comforts are enough to demonstrate your love. Nothing can replace your presence, your hug, your smile, your touch or you!"*
>
> — Denis Waitley, American motivational speaker and author

There's a verse frequently recited when two people make a lifelong commitment to each other. It presents principles to help us understand what love is. I use this verse as a checklist to support and lead me in being loving. As I go through the list, I also ask questions:

- *Love is patient.* Am I being patient?

- *Love is kind.* Am I being kind and considerate?

- *Love does not envy.* Am I pleased for another's good fortune or am I envious and jealous?

- *Love does not boast. It is not proud.* Am I boasting? Am I conceited, arrogant and prideful?

- *Love is not rude, self-seeking or easily angered. It keeps no record of wrongs.* Am I being rude and unmannerly? Am I looking out for only me? Am I becoming angry when I need to be understanding? Am I remembering the past instead of dealing with the now? Am I touchy, fretful or resentful?

- *Love does not delight in evil, but rejoices in the truth.* Am I pleased to see others having troubles? Am I more concerned with retribution and revenge than seeking solutions?

- *Love always protects, always trusts, always hopes and always perseveres.* Do I see the best in others? Am I giving up or responding in a protective, trustful, hopeful and persistent manner?
- *Love never fails.* Do I believe that acting in a loving way never fails?

Acting in a loving way does not always come easily; it takes work, commitment, self-awareness and continual action. It is an act of the will. Acting out of love toward others costs, since it may require us to withhold words we want to say. Love may demand us to respond in ways we do not want to respond. It may ask us to give away what we want to hold onto. To have loving relationships with family members, we must decide to act out of love regardless of how we're treated. The line "Love never fails" in the verse above reminds us that when we continue to act out of love, the situation and the relationship will improve.

Giving love to your family members is healthful for them and for you. Shower **LOL**, **L**ots **O**f **L**ove, on them as you are reminded of James Taylor's lyrics, "Things are gonna work out fine if you only will."

> **"Love is not just a sentiment, not just a feeling, not merely a sort of disposition. Love works; it acts; it does things; and the chief thing it does is to edify, build up, cause growth in each of the persons who engages in it and who is engaged by it."**
>
> — J. Paul Sampley, American theologian

Building Strong Family Relationships

Some of the most rewarding and challenging relationships in our lives can be those with family members. It takes energy, perseverance and time to build strong, healthy and loving family relationships. It takes **L**istening, **O**verlooking, **V**alidating and **E**nergy.

In her book *Twelve Steps to a Compassionate Life*, Karen Armstrong describes how families can be a school for learning compassion.

We learn self-sacrifice because we need to put ourselves to one side to accommodate the needs of other family members. And nearly every day something arises where forgiveness is needed. Armstrong suggests that instead of seeing these tensions as irritants, we view them as opportunities for growth and transformation. To help in this process, ask what makes you proud and happy about your family; what are the ways in which your family nourishes you?

I see family as a *we* thing, not a *me* thing. It's about the people who make up the family unit, not just about one member of the family. In a family, everybody's needs, goals and personalities are important. Every member impacts the others in a family because they are all dependent on each other.

I have a large family. My family of origin and my immediate, or chosen, family come from a base of seven children. I am the second child of parents who immigrated from the Netherlands. They raised four daughters and three sons. Today my family of origin has over forty members. It's still growing. My immediate, or chosen, family, the one my husband and I blended together, has two daughters and five sons. It, too, continues to grow as we bring our children's life partners and our grandchildren into the mix. This dynamic and exceptional blend of family members also includes our in-laws, as well as ex-spouses and their new partners. It brings together a diverse combination of personalities, interests and vibrancy that, in turn, creates interesting challenges in establishing caring and supportive relationships among its members.

The following list is a guide I use regularly to remind myself how family members, including myself, can function as loving members of a family unit. I would say it is a work in progress.

- Our common welfare as a family comes first; personal progress for all family members depends on unity and stability.

- We need a loving higher spirit as the authority of our family; it's not the parent, a spoiled child or my fears that dominate or control our family unit.

- The only requirement for membership in our family is to be part of it; it's not necessary to have straight A's, perfect manners or a charming personality.

- Each of us is encouraged to be an individual and develop our abilities, skills or talents, except when to do so is detrimental to the family as a whole; we try to keep balance in our family.

- I practice self-responsibility myself; I try to encourage and understand my family members, welcoming them and giving them comfort when appropriate.

- I do not meddle, intervene or give unsolicited advice to my adult children lest problems of control, resentment or anger divert us from our primarily loving relationship.

- Each family member needs to be self-supporting to avoid creating dependency.

- My relationships need to remain forever loving, and I may say no as required.

- I do not have to organize or direct our whole family; there may be some who are more responsible than I am.

- I do not need to express my opinion on others' disagreements or take sides, unless I want to be drawn into the middle of their disputes.

- My influence in the family is based on attraction rather than position, and I need to guard with special care the uniqueness of each family member.

- Anonymity limits the glory-seeking, power-seeking, egos and personalities within the family and gives me the courage to be me; I place principles above personalities.

Families include many personality types. Understanding and appreciating the personalities of our loved ones enables us to build stronger family relationships. In their book *Please Understand Me: Character and Temperament Types*, David Keirsey and Marilyn Bates classify and categorize different personality types. They base the various types on the assertion that people's values and personalities differ fundamentally from one another. Their poem "Please Understand Me" expresses, "If I do not want what you want, please try not to tell me that my want is wrong. Or if I believe other than you, at least pause before you correct my view." It articulates a request for others to respect and honor others' emotions, actions, beliefs and wants, even when they are different.

It is important to recognize our differences. There is no right or wrong to them. Stay aware that even though they may not be right for you, they may be right for another. Allowing our life partners, parents, children and all those in our lives to be truly themselves is one of the first steps to understanding them, loving them unconditionally and nurturing our differences.

Myers-Briggs and True Colors workshops give people insights into the different motivations, actions and communication approaches of others. Myers-Briggs is a psychometric questionnaire created to measure people's psychological preferences in the way they perceive the world and make decisions. True Colors is a personality assessment tool designed to help people understand different personality styles and behavioral types. Both are used to improve relationships, communication and self-awareness. Human Metrics is another organization that offers a variety of personality tests that you can try. (Please see appendix III.) Often we are a combination of personality types, usually with one type being more dominant than another.

> *"Whatever the circumstances of your life, the understanding of type can make your perceptions clearer, your judgments sounder, and your life closer to your heart's desire."*
>
> — Isabel Briggs Myers (1897–1980), American psychological theorist and cocreator of the Myers-Briggs Type Indicator

Knowing and accepting family members and others as fundamentally different from us fortifies trust, love and appreciation in our homes. To restate Thomas Merton, "The beginning of love is to let those we love be perfectly themselves, and not to twist them to fit our own image. Otherwise we love only the reflection of ourselves we find in them."

> *"Marriage is just an elaborate game that allows two selfish people to periodically feel that they're not."*
> — Paul Reiser, American comedian, actor, author and musician

Couplehood: Love Is Not Enough

The family unit begins with a couple. Their relationship is the bedrock on which the entire family is built.

Couplehood is a primary source of happiness, sharing and intimacy for many of us. It is a stronghold reminding us we are loved and urging us to love in return. Even though we are individuals in our own right, being part of a couple can often make our lives more enjoyable.

Science shows that committed, healthy relationships increase longevity, reduce blood pressure and even speed up the healing of wounds. But being and staying part of a supportive and healthy couple takes work and commitment.

The rose-colored glasses we often wear when we first fall in love can stop us from clearly seeing our beloved's true character. There is truth to the statement "Love is blind"! In time, the qualities first attracting us to each other may no longer be appealing. Learning to co-exist under one roof can be difficult. For our relationships to work and last "till death do us part" requires the same time, energy and commitment we had for each other when we were dating.

A friend of mine advises family and friends who are considering a long-term couple relationship, "You know what you like about them because that's what attracted you in the first place. Find out what you don't like about them and then ask yourself if you can live with it." My husband says, "It is not only about finding the right person; it's also about being the right person!" Our pastor reiterates the same theme when he says, "For better and for worse for as long as we both shall love is dating, for as long as we both shall live is marriage."

When entering into a long-term relationship, we need to accept the other person for who they are today, not for who we think they will become tomorrow or who we think we can change them into becoming. People tend not to change. Remember to **DETACH**, **D**on't **E**ver **T**hink **A**bout **C**hanging **H**im/**H**er.

A forever loving union is the promise of companionship and mutual commitment between two people as they support each other's physical, emotional and spiritual needs. It is more than a sexual union and more than a financial partnership. When two people come together, their lives blend together in an inseparable way as they become a mixture of each other.

When members of a couple do not work on their relationship, their needs and desires will not be met and stress grows. One of the best ways to keep love alive is to learn to communicate and demonstrate love in a way that's meaningful for each partner. Everyone has different tastes when it comes to cars, movies and music. The same individuality also extends to the way we experience and show love. A love language is the way in which we recognize love. This bias is usually the way we communicate our love to those we love. It is what we are familiar with and respond best to.

In his book *The Five Love Languages: How to Express Heartfelt Commitment to*

> "A relationship is like a garden. If it is to thrive it must be watered regularly. Special care must be given, taking into account the seasons as well as any unpredictable weather. New seeds must be sown and weeds must be pulled."
>
> — John Gray, American counselor, lecturer and author

Your Mate, Dr. Gary Chapman explains five categories in which we express and interpret love:

1. Words of affirmation: Showing love through compliments and affirming statements

2. Quality time: Giving undivided attention, even if it's only twenty minutes at a time

3. Gifts: Giving a gift, whether expensive or not

4. Acts of service: Showing love through actions, such as cooking a meal, cleaning a bathroom or fixing a broken railing

5. Physical touch: Expressing love through physical contact, such as a kiss, a touch, a hug, holding hands or high-fiving

Even though we have a primary love language we respond to, this doesn't mean we won't respond to other love languages. It's important to talk about and understand our partner's preference; otherwise our efforts to express how much we love and care for each other may be futile and frustrating for both parties.

Fundamental personality differences between men and women can either enhance or complicate a couple's relationship. Each has different needs when it comes to building relationships. Dr. John Gray in *Men Are from Mars, Women Are from Venus* highlights basic characteristics each gender needs to receive to build, strengthen and sustain their relationship.

> *"Men and women both need love and both need respect. But the cry from a woman's deepest soul is to be loved and the cry from a man's deepest soul is to be respected."*
>
> — Dr. Emerson Eggerichs, American counselor, speaker and author

What Women and Men Want in a Relationship	
Women	**Men**
Caring	Trust
Understanding	Acceptance
Admiration	Appreciation
Devotion	Respect
Validation	Approval
Reassurance	Encouragement

Learning to understand and know how to meet your partner's needs is an ongoing process. Those who do couplehood **BEST** know they need to continually

- **B**less one another with praise, privately and publicly;
- **E**dify and **E**ncourage each other;
- **S**hare thoughts and feelings, big and small; and
- **T**ouch tenderly, lovingly and respectfully.

Another simple acronym to consider in regards to building strong and loving couple relationships is **CAT**. We can enhance our relationship with our beloved through

- **C**ommunication: Continually interacting with each other;
- **A**utonomy: Remaining independent; and

"Healthy love can't be demanded nor taken for granted. It can only be a continuing give-and-take exchange and dialogue between two independent persons who share many values and responsibilities, yet still feel a childlike magic with each other."

— Denis Waitley, American motivational speaker and author

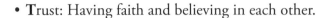

- **T**rust: Having faith and believing in each other.

As time passes, the familiarity that comes with a lifelong commitment may cause you to forget the feelings of love and refreshment you shared at the beginning of your relationship. You can continue to refresh each other with an encouraging word, an unexpected gift or a change of pace. A surprise call or note can be refreshing. Holding off discussions about your frustrations creates trust and understanding. Taking an annual retreat together, perhaps with a facilitator or marriage-enrichment group, is another way to sustain, refresh and strengthen couplehood. Continue to create a relationship where both partners find support, safety and peace of mind.

As an added note, many women suffer with premenstrual syndrome (PMS), a collection of physical and emotional symptoms related to their menstrual cycle. The American College of Obstetricians and Gynecologists estimates that over eighty percent of menstruating women experience at least one PMS symptom as part of their monthly cycle.

A woman's PMS symptoms vary in degree and severity from cycle to cycle. In a male/female partnership, it is wise for both partners to remain cognizant of these times as the mood-related symptoms can have an effect on their relationship. These symptoms include anger and irritability, anxiety, tension, depression, crying, oversensitivity and mood swings. Inability to sleep and increased tiredness can also impact the severity of these symptoms. As a nurse, I spent many years working night shifts and became very aware of the impact of PMS. When my PMS symptoms were added to lack of sleep and stress at home, I was not easy to live with.

In addition, as the female partner heads into menopause, it is wise to remain aware of the impact of its mood-related symptoms. The woman can work to clarify the source of her irritability and moodiness. The man can learn to overlook and forgive these behaviors and not take them personally.

Intimacy in Couplehood

A vital component between couples is intimacy, which develops when two people open their inner selves to each other. The sharing of thoughts, dreams and hopes is important, but we also need to share our fears, experiences and shortcomings, along with our regrets and feelings, while trusting our partner will continue to accept and love us.

Think of intimacy as **in-to-me-see**. It requires openness and vulnerability as we allow our partner to see us for who we truly are. To maintain **in-to-me-see** in your relationship, consider the following five areas:

1. Intellectual intimacy: Sharing and discussing thoughts helps our partner get a sense of what makes us tick. Whether it's our favorite breakfast cereal, the cost of natural gas or people who laugh at their own jokes, every thought we have reveals something about us.

2. Emotional intimacy: Discussing our emotions and feelings and the reasons behind them requires vulnerability. We need to trust our partner will not withdraw from us or condemn us as they discover more about us.

3. Social intimacy: Doing things together, whether with a group or on our own, continues our dating life.

4. Spiritual intimacy: Sharing our beliefs and spirituality leads to respect and understanding as we discover how experiences, philosophies and interpretations affect each other. Participating in spiritual practices together can draw couples closer together.

5. Physical intimacy: Expressing love physically requires understanding the differences between what men and women require sexually. The emotional aspect of sex tends to be important to women, whereas the physical is important to most men.

Physical or sexual intimacy is intended to give pleasure. Learning, understanding and fulfilling each other's sexual preferences and needs helps us give pleasure to our partner. It is a critical component of a healthy, happy and loving relationship. Sex is the glue of intimacy, creating a strong bond between two people. Orgasm is the most biochemical bonding event that humans can experience. It relieves stress and brings two people into a closeness that cannot be achieved in any other way.

Sex is a gift for a couple's mutual enjoyment. It's not intended to be boring, lifeless, pleasureless or dull. When it becomes routine, temptations may entice partners to be unfaithful to each other for excitement and pleasure elsewhere. However, being faithful to your partner assures the greatest fulfillment for both partners.

Sexual unfaithfulness damages and breaks the spark in a relationship. It breaks the bond. It leads to an inability to feel fully committed, to feel sexual desire and to trust. Sexual unfaithfulness destroys family life, erodes our ability to love and degrades us. It turns people into objects. It can also lead to disease and unwanted children.

Sexual unfaithfulness includes physical affairs and virtual affairs. Visiting online sex sites displaces the intended purpose of a loving sexual relationship as it dislocates sex from intimacy, training our minds to exalt what is least important about someone, while ignoring what is most important. It is also strongly addicting. Remain a loving partner and look to your partner for satisfaction and companionship. Don't endanger yourself or your family's health and security.

Advice from Marriage Counselors

Thirty-eight percent of Canadian marriages and almost fifty percent in the United States end in divorce. Divorce costs billions of dollars in legal and real estate fees alone, not to mention the psychological toll on the couple, the children, the extended family and friends. It also costs our places of employment and society. Divorce is a loss to everyone it touches, a loss that results in feelings of grief and emotional turmoil, just like the grief we experience when a loved one dies.

My husband and I have both been divorced and, along with our children, extended family and friends, we have experienced its unpleasant consequences. Some of these consequences may continue for years, and others may endure forever. Divorce, a choice not made lightly, impacts many people's lives. Its fallout creates turmoil for all those involved. Seeking new ways and putting effort into maintaining a loving relationship with each other is often a better choice.

Marriage counselors suggest that with the right communication tools, realistic expectations and a lifetime of elbow grease, most marriages can last and be fun. The following list, adapted from a 2010 issue of *Reader's Digest*, highlights advice marriage counselors give to married couples, or to anyone considering a lifelong relationship:

- There is no such thing as Mr. or Ms. Right. Good relationships are the result of effort and dedication; they do not just happen.

- Talk isn't cheap; it's your most valuable investment. Open and regular communication is key as it creates connection, empathy and intimacy.

- A relationship is like a car; you need to change the oil regularly. It is important to have the how-are-we-doing conversation every three months—no matter how long you've been married. This ensures issues or grievances are addressed, heading off trouble before the problem becomes too big to handle. Make time for it. Mark it on the calendar.

- Being emotional is better than being rational. Relationships are by their very nature emotional, not rational, so talk about how you feel. Say, "This is what I fear," "This is what I need" or "This is what hurt my feelings." Then use the facts to make rational decisions.

- *No one wins unless you both do.* When it comes to feelings, nobody's right or wrong. Going into situations with a win-lose attitude leads to both losing.

- How you feel is up to you; don't blame others for how you feel. Your feelings are your own. It's not what happens or how you feel about it, it's what you make it mean.

- Women aren't from Venus and men aren't from Mars; males and females tend to be more similar than different.

- When you argue, it should be all about you. You are the expert on your thoughts and feelings, no one else is. Stay with the **I Over You**, or **IOU**, language, *I* think, *I* feel and *I* need.

- It's not about money; it's about what you think about money. Money is one of three things couples fight about most. Sex and the division of labor are the others. Money, like sex, is about trust. Every person has a financial style, and neither is right or wrong. Sorting out what each person is comfortable with is key. Consider having three bank accounts—his, hers and ours.

- Sex: It's mostly about talking—and fun. Most couples struggle with low or mismatched sexual desire. For dual-career couples, sometimes referred to as **DINS, D**ual **I**ncome, **N**o **S**ex, low libido is more common than erectile dysfunction or lack of orgasms. Discuss sex openly and at an appropriate time. Remember, sex is relationship glue. It's healthful, a great coping mechanism and an effective stress-management tool.

Marriage counselors also stress that time spent together needs to be playful, intimate and easy. Couplehood is meant to be a fun, life-long journey with many conversations.

Taking Time for Ourselves in Our Relationships

No matter how wonderful togetherness feels, it is crucial to take time for ourselves. There is simply no person who can fulfill all our needs. We need to maintain that responsibility ourselves.

Often a partner will give up a favorite hobby, sport or pastime in order to devote more time and energy to the relationship. But giving up interests and the things we do to nurture ourselves eventually leads to relationship stress, miscommunication, resentment and emotional pain. It also takes away some of the interesting aspects about ourselves that first attracted our partners to us.

Independence is good for both partners, no matter how close you may be. Taking time to be alone, to pursue other interests and go out with your friends encourages your partner to do the same. When you reconnect, you feel renewed and excited to share your experience and to be with each other.

As part of a couple, we depend on each other. If one does not take proper care of themselves, it impacts the other. As adults, we do not need someone to look after us. I say to my husband, "I'll take care of me for you and you take care of you for me."

Taking responsibility for ourselves in our relationships also involves taking care of our physical needs with proper nutrition, exercise and regular health checkups. Also, maintaining our looks with proper grooming and hygiene keeps us feeling good about ourselves, and it keeps our partner attracted to us.

Taking care of our bodies is important for our future. Many partners pass away prematurely because of poor health habits, leaving the other alone. Their beloved and their family members are no longer able to enjoy and spend time with them. A relationship intended to last many years is cut short because one neglected their responsibility to care for themselves. By doing our part, we can increase our chances to be with our partner in our "golden years."

It Takes a Village to Raise a Child

Just as our family component is important to our balance wheels of health and well-being, the same is true with our children's balance wheels. In fact, our satisfaction with family has a strong impact on how satisfied our children will be with their family component as well as with all six components of their balance wheel of health and well-being.

> *"The country clubs, the cars, the boats, your assets may be ample, but the best inheritance you can leave your kids is to be a good example."*
>
> — Barry Spilchuk, Canadian speaker and trainer

Children are an asset to our families, our communities and our world. They enrich our lives and teach us many things about life and ourselves. Children do not belong only to their parents or their families; they also belong to the world, to the future.

Many of us are given the privilege and opportunity to raise children, or to be involved in raising and guiding children for a period of time until it's time to let them go free into the world to build their own lives. Raising children is a huge responsibility. It is probably the most important and difficult task we will undertake.

> *"There are only two lasting bequests we can hope to give our children. One of these is roots; the other is wings."*
>
> — Hodding Carter II (1907–1972), American journalist and author

Raising children requires a great deal of energy, time and commitment. It is not just about being custodial and seeing to their physical health and well-being. It means teaching, loving and conveying respect; opening the doors to exploration; and standing back and waiting. Raising children means supporting them only for as long as necessary for them to become independent. When we raise children, we teach them about loving, relating to and forgiving others as we open up their opportunities for intimacy with a range of people from many walks of life. Believing that one or two parents can provide all this to a child is limiting—it can completely overwhelm even the best of us.

Whether you raise your children with a partner or as a single parent, there is great truth in the ancient African proverb "It takes a village to raise a child." Parenting is easier and better when we are part of a network of other people and/or a community.

Just as our children need their families and other people to support and love them, they also need the diversity that comes from experiencing different activities, environments, cultures and people helping them

> *"Two parents can't raise a child any more than one. We need a whole community— everybody—to raise a child."*
>
> — Toni Morrison, American author

to understand the complexities and the simplicities of life. They need to be a part of a loving, caring community. That community can be a traditional setting with a mother, father, siblings, grandparents, aunts, uncles and cousins. It can be the neighborhood, schools, sport or church groups or a combination of them all. Many people are involved with parents in raising a child to be a healthy, confident, self-supporting and caring adult.

I have three children. The difference between the youngest and the oldest is eleven years. Within that time frame, I have noticed changes in the way parents raise their children. Author and speaker Elisabeth Elliot wrote, "Parents used to want their children to be good, and as a result of being good they were usually happy. Now there has been a subtle turn—parents want their children to be happy."

But oftentimes, being happy does not include being good, whereas when we provide our children with opportunities for being good, happiness looks after itself. When we teach children to care for themselves and to serve and care for the needs of others, they become responsible adults. Raising a child in a healthful, supportive environment ensures he or she will be healthy in body, mind and soul. That way our children become adults who benefit their own families and the world around them.

As well, children need to develop trust in those who provide guidance to them. Even though they may test the boundaries, they still need to feel safe and secure. If parents are not consistent with discipline and correction, boundaries will be bent and broken, leading to insecurity and confusion. As author and speaker Stuart Briscoe says, "Be firm, be fair, be fun!"

> *"It is easier to build strong children than to repair broken men."*
> — Frederick Douglass (1818–1895), American social reformer, author and statesman

Parental responsibility often requires more than our time, energy and love. To be effective in our role, we may need to seek help from parenting courses or books on parenting. There are many qualified people and books we can go to. In his book *The World's Easiest Guide to Family Relationships*, Dr. Chapman highlights what he calls "an old family recipe" that lists five ingredients he believes are needed for the development of healthy, independent children within the family unit:

1. An attitude of service: Household chores such as folding laundry, washing dishes and making beds, along with mopping floors, feeding pets, making meals and washing cars, provide numerous shared service opportunities. When we train and encourage children to do and complete mundane and often thankless tasks, we provide them with a sense of satisfaction and accomplishment. By teaching them the value of responsibility and how to work well with others, we help them identify some of their talents and strengths.

2. Intimacy between parents or partners: The parental relationship sets an example of how to interact and be good future parents and partners. Showing children healthy forms of

intellectual, emotional, social, spiritual and physical intimacy between parents is vital.

3. Parents who teach and train: Learning how to survive and thrive in this world involves teaching them through instruction, encouragement, correction and affirmation. Training involves showing them what to do or guiding them in positive ways. Demonstrating values such as honesty, hard work and courage equips them to respond positively to fear, anger and disappointment and builds their characters. Children watch adults for clues on how to live their own lives. We need to ensure our actions match our words.

4. Children who obey and honor their parents: Obedience is learned by following the rules. All actions have consequences—positive actions bring positive consequences and negative actions bring negative consequences. Rules and boundaries are a necessary part of living in unity and harmony; without them there's no structure or security. Establishing rules, setting or allowing appropriate consequences and administering discipline are all part of obedience.

5. Fathers who are loving leaders: Even though there are many families with wonderful, strong woman as the only leader, Chapman states male leadership is important. I tend to agree. When I was a single parent, there were many times during the day-to-day raising of my children when I was aware of how the assistance of a loving and supportive father figure would have enhanced their upbringing. Male leadership helps demonstrate

> *"Fathers, do not irritate and provoke your children to anger, do not exasperate them to resentment, but rear them tenderly in training and discipline."*
> — Ephesians 6:4

male responsibility, dependability and commitment to family. As leaders, a father needs to be active in parenting, make time to be with his children, provide for and protect them, engage them in conversation, play with them and teach them positive values, all while loving them unconditionally. This helps prepare children for bringing up their own families.

Time and the Family Meal

Giving time is one way to show love to family members. Time with one another allows us to experience the joy of being with those we love. There is no substitute for taking time to be together.

We all live busy lives, so making time for pleasant memories must be arranged in advance. We are given only 168 hours a week, and just as our paychecks need to be budgeted and spent wisely to cover all our needs, our time needs to be spent wisely. After we have slept, bathed, dressed, eaten, worked, commuted, responded to messages on our social media devices and taken care of groceries and home mainte-nance, how much discretionary time is left for relationships? We may need to work at creating adequate quality time with our families.

"If you want your children to turn out well, spend twice as much time with them and half as much money on them."

— Abigail Van Buren, American advice columnist

Family members need time together to be and stay connected. One of the most accessible tools for bringing families closer is mealtime. It's a place to gather and exchange information about everyone's day and share its victories and heartbreaks with the people who care about us.

Even though eating together is meant to be a time of connection, mealtime com-petes with after-school and after-work activities, electronic entertainment, dual-career households and many other distractions. Many homes become like boarding houses, with family members passing each other on their way to individual activities. With a million voices shouting in our ears, getting together at the same time and in the same place can become a monumental task.

A 2008 report for the Society for Research in Child Development in the United States showed that children who regularly engage with their parents around the meal table have larger vocabularies, make better grades, eat more fruits and vegetables and are less likely to experiment with drugs and premarital sex.[2] Putting the effort into arranging these get-togethers is worth it.

Child-development experts say children, especially teens, communicate better with their parents when they have a peripheral activity to remove some of the pressure. At the table or the kitchen counter, buttering a slice of bread, refilling a glass of milk or scooping a forkful of salad provides the perfect distraction for children to share their day, their concerns and themselves with us. It provides us with an opportunity to connect and listen, while they feel comfortable enough to open up and share.

Once communication is flowing, there is an opportunity to process the experiences of the day with family members, to help gain perspective and to consider things in a holistic context. Mealtime is about connecting as well as encouraging, exhorting and debriefing together—discussing what the world has thrown at each of us that day.

Sharing good times together is like making deposits into an emotional bank account. Every time we have a positive exchange with someone, we make a "trust" deposit into our relational bank account, building up a reserve. Conversely, when we have a negative exchange, our relationship reserve is depleted by whatever crisis we are experiencing. A history of mealtimes together with positive communication

---

2. Barbara H. Fiese and Marlene Schwartz, "Reclaiming the Family Table: Mealtimes and Child Health and Wellbeing," *Social Policy Report* 22, no. 4 (2008), http://familyresiliency.illinois.edu/policy/documents/SRCDReclaimingthe FamilyDinnerTable_2008.pdf.

is invaluable during difficult times as we will have amassed a healthy "account balance" from which to draw.

Here are some **TIP**s **T**o **I**mprove your **P**erformance for making mealtime a priority in building family bonds and memories:

- Aim to share mealtimes together three times a week. Get a solid commitment from each member for those times. If this is too much, start with one.
- If someone is late, wait.
- Keep mealtimes stress-free, relaxed and fun. Be positive. Don't choose this time to discipline or complain.
- Ban cell phones, hand-held video devices, TV and the telephone.
- Take turns preparing the meal and setting the table, as well as clearing and washing dishes.
- Share news about your day and ask open-ended questions to get others talking about their day.
- Practice active listening—know when to talk and when to listen.
- Be creative, flexible and open to discussion topics and conversation flow; be the same with the types of food prepared and how it's served.
- Teach, don't preach.
- Any mealtime works—Saturday brunch, Sunday lunch, even breakfast.

How Do You Communicate?

When a family member acts out, they do so for a reason—something has caused them to feel disrespected. Often our words and actions cause family members to feel disrespected. Resentment, name calling and jealousy create frustration or anger, which leads to outbursts that can usually be traced to someone feeling hurt because they did not feel important. Whether they're right or wrong, the only way to fix the situation is to show them they are cared about.

Loving communication is critical to building relationships, but true communication is different from talking. It is verbal and nonverbal. Talking is often a one-way activity, whereas true communication involves the art of speaking, listening, interpreting and confirming people's dreams, fears, thoughts and aspirations. What we say and how we say it creates emotions and thoughts in others. A kind word helps people; negative words hurt—sometimes for a very long time.

The proverb "The tongue has the power of life and death, and those who love to talk will have to eat their own words" holds a lot of wisdom. Another proverb says "He who guards his lips guards his life, but he who speaks rashly will come to ruin." Our words can heal or tear down.

The saying "Sticks and stones may break my bones, but words will never hurt me" is a fallacy. Words do, in fact, hurt us deeply. Communicating with positive versus negative language keeps our balance wheels of health and well-being inflated. To build healthy relationships with our loved ones, we need to train ourselves to control the words we speak to avoid saying hurtful and negative things. When difficult conversations happen, it is important that we have developed the habit of curbing our tongue. We can't take back our negative words once said. Talking too much, saying things we should not say and sharing the confidences of others damages relationships. Gossiping, complaining and speaking harshly are all negative communication styles.

More than what we say, our body language demonstrates how we really feel. Nonverbal communication includes posture, gestures, facial expressions, attentiveness and tone of voice. To be an effective communicator, we need to ensure our actions align with our words.

Do you cross your arms, roll your eyes, tap your fingers or look at your watch when you speak with someone? To communicate effectively, look people in the eye, stop what you are doing and put away your cell phone, turn off the TV and turn down the music.

Consider the tone and sincerity of what you are saying. At what volume and speed do you speak? Do you cut people off in mid-sentence? Are you almost yelling? What words of endearment do you use—"sweetheart," "honey" or "sugar plum"? Or do you use "stupid," "idiot" and "dummy"? Is your tone of voice gentle and reassuring or harsh and accusing? Do you speak to people the way you want to be spoken to?

Do you make promises you don't keep? Are you critical, condescending or sarcastic toward those you speak with? Some of us become masters at the art of bludgeoning with bitter words and shredding others with scorn. Some speak arrogantly to show others they can't be hurt or to relieve pent-up feelings.

When we use negative tones in our communication, we often unintentionally lash out and hurt those we love. Consider the word *sarcasm*. Sarcasm comes from the Greek verb *sarkazein*, which means "to tear flesh." When you use sarcasm, it might feel fun or smart, but you may be creating deep wounds that are slow to heal.

The way we communicate and respond to our loved ones can increase stress levels.

We need to learn to attack the problem and not the person. As parents, partners and children, expressing our love through positive communication styles builds confidence and self-esteem in our loved ones while reducing stress. Every type of verbal and nonverbal communication we deliver has the potential to be a brick to build enduring relationships or a bulldozer to push relationships apart. The words and actions of communication are like seeds; they carry creative or destructive power to produce either a good or bad crop in our lives and in the lives of those we love.

The most important communication skill is to **listen**. Be quick to listen and slow to speak. Consider how the letters in **listen** are the same as the letters in **silent**. We need to be **silent** so we can **listen** to others speak and truly hear what they say. We have two ears to hear and one mouth to speak. Seek first to understand by really listening.

Be cautious when choosing words that may cause people to give up or quit. Negative words destroy the human spirit—low self-esteem, self-worth and depression can be created by a flow of words that consistently hurt, break down or control others. Our mouths and words are the vehicles we use to communicate what is in our hearts. They need to be tools that heal, restore and uplift and not tools that lead to conflict.

Here are some more **TIP**s **T**o **I**mprove your **P**erformance in communication:

- **THINK** before you speak. Ensure what you say is **T**houghtful, **H**onest, **I**ntelligent, **N**ecessary and **K**ind.

- Before making important decisions or discussing important topics with others, **HALT**. If you are **H**ungry, **A**ngry, **L**onely or **T**ired, address these issues first, before you respond or take action.

- Responding to family members with love and respect builds self-esteem and enhances your relationships. The **BEST** approach is to **B**less them with praise, **E**dify and **E**ncourage them and **S**hare your feelings and thoughts in a gentle way while you spend adequate quality **T**ime with them.

Setting Boundaries

Dr. Henry Cloud and Dr. John Townsend write about setting boundaries with the people in our lives to avoid or minimize the intrusion of unhealthful influences. They help us distinguish between what is our responsibility and what is not. Boundaries guard our hearts and help us fence in what nurtures us, while keeping out what will harm us. They keep the good in and the bad out.

In their book *Boundaries: When to Say YES, When to Say NO to Take Control of Your Life*, Dr. Cloud and Dr. Townsend teach that boundaries are not impenetrable walls. They need gates to help us establish effective and healthy relationships. These portals are to be open when we are safe and closed when we are attacked, demeaned or overwhelmed.

Setting and honoring boundaries in relationships keeps us from being taken advantage of, but they don't help us when they are too loose or too rigid. They need to be flexible so they are good for everyone in the relationship. However, they need to be consistent to be effective. Healthy boundaries demonstrate self-respect while still respecting others, and the responses to our boundaries help us evaluate the quality of our relationships.

> "He that respects himself is safe from others, he wears a coat of mail that none can pierce."
>
> — Henry Wadsworth Longfellow (1807–1882), American poet

Do you respect other people's boundaries, and do the people in your life respect your boundaries? Do you respect your own boundaries?

It can be challenging to define and establish healthy boundaries for ourselves, as the process requires clear thinking and communication. The most basic boundary-setting word is no. Remember, *no is a complete sentence, not requiring a defense or justification.*

Not everyone will agree with your choices or boundaries, nor will they share your values. As you take responsibility to honor yourself, you'll make choices and set boundaries with your best interests in mind. In doing so, a question you may consider asking yourself is, "In light of my past experience, my future hopes and dreams and where I am right now, what are the best boundaries or limits to set in place?"

Others may not understand the choices you make, but they need to respect them. If you allow your boundaries to be repeatedly violated, you become a volunteer in an unhealthy relationship, not a victim. It's your responsibility to build relationships with people who are affirming and trustworthy, so limit your exposure to those who are not. You demonstrate dignity and respect for yourself when you honor your values, choices and boundaries. You demonstrate dignity and respect for others when you honor their boundaries. A healthy relationship is a two-way street, where each person respects the other's right-of-way.

A Wounded Child

It has been said that society's history, politics, success or lack of success can always be made clearer when we look at the childhoods of the individuals involved. Our greatest needs are when we are young. These needs include safety, attention, guidance, acceptance, freedom, tolerance, validation, trust, nurturing and unconditional love. Rarely are we raised by parents capable of providing or meeting all our needs. We have all felt hurt, rejection, neglect and unfairness of some kind.

Inner child is a concept used in psychology to denote the childlike aspect of our psyches. The term is used to address our childhood experiences and their remaining effects. It also refers to the emotional memory and experiences stored in our brains.

Carl Jung, a Swiss psychologist and psychiatrist, referred to the concept as the *divine child*; Emmet Fox, a new-thought spiritual leader, called it the *wonder child*; Charles Whitfield, a medical doctor and psychotherapist, called it the *child within*; and other psychotherapists call it the *true self*. John Bradshaw, an educator and self-help leader, modified the concept to the *wounded inner child*.

> *"Whatever is denied conscious access continues to influence the individual anyhow— but via unconscious processes."*
>
> — Carl Jung (1875–1961), Swiss psychologist and psychiatrist

When we do not explore our feelings, the unconscious processes can have a significant impact on our sense of self, our adult relationships and our lives. Our emotional wounds are stored up as energy in our bodies. When not processed, they can have a great effect on us. Dr. Whitfield said, "When we are not allowed to remember, to express our feelings and to grieve or mourn our losses or trauma, whether real or threatened, through the free expression of our *child within*, we become ill." This "illness" can and does take on many forms.

You may have a lost, frightened and frozen child inside of you. You may be carrying wounds around with you and unknowingly pass them on to your children, like an inheritance, wounding them and continuing the cycle. *To truly love the adult you are, you need to own the child you were.* Searching out and getting acquainted with your inner child may enhance your adult life and your ability to be a loving parent.

When children have been sexually abused, it is understandable to assume they will experience many problems later in life. It is also understandable that when children are physically abused, they may go on to physically abuse their own children. Emotional abuse is just as destructive and painful as physical and sexual abuse. Yet some may not understand its impact. If you are hit by a Volkswagen, and another person is hit by a Mack truck, both of you will experience pain, hurt and injuries. Do not minimize the impact of your experiences. Pain is pain. Your pain, hurt and wounds need to be addressed and they need to be healed.

A number of indications that may enlighten you to the fact that you carry wounds from your childhood include

- constant mistrust about life, constant feelings of shame and doubt and a constant need to please people;
- constant turmoil in relationships or lack of healthy, intimate relationships;
- persistent feelings of loneliness, isolation and separation from everyone;
- persistent need to judge, criticize, condemn and blame yourself or others for your problems;

- fear of intimacy;

- trust and codependency issues;

- problems with authority and hierarchy;

- holding onto anger, resentment, jealousy, fear and guilt;

- a strong attitude of "what's in this for me?" in everything you do;

- strong reactions to situations that usually don't bother others;

- feeling responsible for other people's misery or feeling responsible for your parents' failure in marriage and/or their careers; and

- unconsciously acting as a spouse to an unhappy and emotionally wounded parent.

John Bradshaw is a major figure in the field of recovery and dysfunctional families. He believes wounds received in childhood can continue to contaminate the lives of adults and are the root cause of many of the problems we face as adults. In his book *Homecoming: Reclaiming and Championing Your Inner Child*, he includes a wounded-child questionnaire. Bradshaw suggests that answering yes to ten or more of the sixty questions he lists indicates that you need to do some serious work.

Being aware of what constitutes emotional abuse toward children may help to ensure you don't have a wounded inner child within you wreaking havoc in your adult life. Emotional abuse to children includes the following:

> *"In reclaiming and championing your wounded inner child, you give him the positive, unconditional acceptance that he craves. That will release him to recognize and love others for who they are."*
>
> — John Elliot Bradshaw, American educator, counselor, speaker and author

- Shaming: Repressing or forcing children to adapt to specific behaviors and the views of parents

- Not allowing a child to just be: Stunting or denying children the opportunity to express their true feelings or natural state

- Being inflexible: Rigid or inflexible rules

- Being repressive: Protectiveness or instilling fear that the world around them is a dangerous place

- Being emotionally absent: Not spending quality time with children

There are many more ways children can be wounded by a caregiver. Coming to terms with issues and wounds from childhood and seeking help ensures you do not pass on your legacy to your own children. Doing so benefits you and others. It can show you a life free from emotions that may be driven by the three-year-old child inside you.

Here are some **TIP**s to heal your wounded inner child:

- Seek effective counseling and/or share with others in a safe environment.

- Discover your hidden negative beliefs.

- Take responsibility for your own feelings and emotions and allow yourself to feel and experience them.

- Know you are not responsible for the failures or misery of your parents or of others.

- Find time to be alone to feel calm and nurtured.

- Seek and use quality self-help CDs and literature.

- Practice meditation and visualization techniques or write about your feelings and experiences.

- Use positive affirmations.

A Family Disease

Boundaries are often crossed in families. Perhaps out of ignorance. Perhaps due to old familiar habits. It's difficult not to cross some boundaries when you live at close quarters with each other. Maintaining healthy boundaries when you live with active addiction is even more difficult.

Addiction is usually defined as physical and psychological dependence on psychoactive substances such as alcohol, tobacco, heroin and other drugs that cross the blood-brain barrier once ingested and alter the chemical environment of the brain. Addiction is the continued involvement with a substance or activity despite the negative consequences associated with it.

Those living and dealing with various forms of addictions are everywhere. They can be our friends, neighbors or fellow church members. They can be our medical, financial or legal professionals.

Addictions result in poor physical health for the one addicted. They also cause problems in families and relationships. They lead to stress, causing everyday life to become a constant struggle. When there is addiction in our homes and families, there is uneasiness, conflict and oftentimes havoc. It can be crazy making. Addictions affect all who are touched by it.

I cannot say if one addiction causes more turmoil inside the family unit than another, but I have chosen to focus on alcohol addiction because of my personal experience living with someone with active alcoholism, knowing that all addictions operate in a similar manner, and that for every person suffering with this disease, a minimum of six others are affected.

Many people acknowledge that alcoholism is a disease, but they may not know it as a *family* disease. It's a disorder that affects every member of the family, often without their realizing it. It affects them emotionally, physically and spiritually. How people deal with its effects varies. The following are common themes expressed by those who

> "Any family, wife and children, who have had to live with an alcoholic for ten or fifteen years, are bound to be rather neurotic and distorted themselves. They just can't help it."
>
> — William Griffith Wilson (1895–1971), American cofounder of Alcoholics Anonymous

have lived with the disease; they demonstrate how the addiction has affected them. As you read through them, feel free to change the word *alcoholism* to another addiction, or just use the word *addiction*.

- Alcoholism is a thief. It pickpockets job opportunities, close relationships and our physical safety. It robs us of those we love and, in some cases, it eventually steals a life.

- Alcoholism stole trust and security from my childhood, leading me to grow up feeling like a counterfeit adult. I was someone who looked and acted well adjusted on the outside, but on the inside I was lost, frightened and confused.

- I struggle with the effects of alcoholism, even though I don't drink. Because I needed to survive constant crises, broken promises, embarrassments and lost dreams, I chose to deny the truth about my situation. Because of the stubborn self-reliance I developed, it wiped out the guidance and comfort available to me from loving family and friends. In time, I became resentful and lost the love and goodwill of others. Due to obsessive worry, I was unwilling to accept and enjoy life.

Children who live with alcoholism often have more problems dealing with the nondrinking parent than they do with the drinking parent. The nondrinking parent may say, "I don't have a problem! He's the alcoholic! He's the one who causes the problems and is in trouble all the time." There may be truth to those comments, but often the drinking parent is the one who at least behaves in a predictable fashion, whereas the nondrinking parent does not.

Children and teenagers learn to read the alcoholic like a book. They know when it's the right time to ask for extra money or to go somewhere with friends. They learn the routines of the alcoholic and when it's time to get out of the way and make themselves scarce. But they never know where the nondrinking parent will be coming from next. One minute this parent is screaming at the alcoholic, threatening them with everything from divorce to death. The next minute they may be compassionately rescuing the drinking parent from the consequences of the latest drinking episode, dutifully cleaning up the messes, making excuses for them and accepting an increasing degree of unhealthful and unacceptable behavior. Minutes later, the nondrinking parent may be screaming at the children, taking their anger out on the innocent.

The disease of alcoholism affects the nondrinking partner's life, attitude and thinking perhaps more dramatically than it affects the drinking partner, but the nondrinking partner doesn't even realize it as it creeps up on them so slowly.

If you put a frog into a pan of boiling water, it'll jump out lickety-split. But if you put the frog into a pan of water that's the frog's body temperature, and then slowly turn up the heat, the frog will stay in the water even to the point of boiling to death. The frog doesn't notice the gradual change.

Living with alcoholism works the same way. The heat is slowly and repeatedly turned up, but nobody notices; it's a cunning and baffling progressive disease. It may start out with casually accepting unacceptable behavior: "Oh, he didn't mean that. He just had too much to drink last night." A few years later the behavior has grown more and more intolerable, but it's still being accepted and has become "normal."

The nondrinking partner ends up with chaos in their home that a few years before would have been unacceptable and unthinkable. As the behavior becomes routine, the last thing that would occur to them is to pick up the phone to get help. They've slowly been drawn into thinking the alcoholic should be protected, and they have learned to cover for them. They lie for them and have learned to keep secrets, no matter how bad the chaos and insanity have become.

Few who have been affected by the disease of alcoholism realize that by protecting the alcoholic, they make it easier for them to continue drinking and progress in their downward spiral. Rather than helping the alcoholic and themselves, the nondrinking partner enables the drinking partner to get worse. The disease continues to progress for the alcoholic until they are ready to reach out and get help for themselves. But family members can begin to recover, whether the alcoholic is still drinking or not, by picking up the phone and asking for help.

There are various centers that offer addiction counseling and support to those who have been affected by it. There are also many twelve-step programs around the world that help those with addictions and those who live with or have lived with someone else's addiction. (Please see appendix III.)

Abusive Relationships

Domestic violence, elder abuse, sexual abuse and other forms of abuse can happen to anyone, regardless of their age, gender or strength. Yet the problem, as with addictions, is often overlooked, excused or denied. This is especially true when the abuse is psychological rather than physical. Emotional and financial abuses are often minimized, but they leave deep and lasting scars. Any form of abuse crosses personal boundaries.

Noticing and acknowledging warning signs and symptoms of family violence and abuse is the first step to ending it. The following questionnaire lists warning signs and descriptions of abuse. The more times you answer yes, the more likely you are in an abusive relationship.

Signs That You Are in an Abusive Relationship

Your Inner Thoughts and Feelings	Your Partner's or Family Member's Belittling Behavior
Do you • feel afraid of your partner or family member much of the time? • avoid certain topics out of fear of angering your partner or family member? • feel that you can't do anything right for your partner or family member? • believe you deserve to be hurt or mistreated? • wonder if you are the one who is crazy? • feel emotionally numb or helpless?	Does your partner or family member • humiliate or yell at you? • criticize you or put you down? • treat you so badly you're embarrassed in the company of friends or family? • ignore you or put down your opinions or accomplishments? • blame you for their abusive behavior? • see you as property or a sex object rather than as a person?

Your Partner's or Family Member's Violent Behavior or Threats	Your Partner's or Family Member's Controlling Behavior
Does your partner or family member • have a bad and unpredictable temper? • hurt you or threaten to hurt or kill you? • threaten to take your children away or harm them? • threaten to commit suicide if you leave? • force you to have sex? • destroy your belongings?	Does your partner or family member • act excessively jealous and possessive? • control where you go or what you do? • keep you from seeing your friends or other family members? • limit your access to money, the phone or the car? • constantly check up on you?

There may come a time when a person who has been abused makes up their mind and says, "Nobody is ever going to push me around again. Nobody is going to tell me what to do. From now on, I'm going to look out for myself and make my own decisions."

But once people manage to leave an abusive or highly dysfunctional environment, the effects of that environment don't suddenly disappear.

Frequently, the person who has been abused becomes willful, stubborn and rebellious because they were controlled and manipulated for years by someone who was meant to love them.

Hurting, wounded people are often drawn to other hurting, wounded people. Individuals from long-term abuse often partner with or marry someone who also experienced long-term abuse, leading to the truth behind the phrase "Hurt people hurt people." The cycle of abuse continues. Children often pick up abusive tendencies and pass them on to the next generation.

Abusive cycles will not be broken until someone decides to stop them, and then they reach out to receive appropriate help. Awareness must be achieved and acted on in order to begin to make wiser and more healthful life choices. Calling your local helpline listed in your phone book or on the Internet will open the door to the needed assistance. (Please see appendix III.)

Forgive Them!

"The weak can never forgive. Forgiveness is the attribute of the strong."

— Mahatma Gandhi (1869–1948), Indian political and spiritual leader

Addiction and abuse cause hurt, pain and misery, often coming from those we love and those who love us. In response to this violation, the ability to forgive is the most important asset we can acquire. As we deal with the difficult and challenging relationships that deteriorate the quality of our lives, holding onto past hurts and pains hardens our hearts. Carrying these heavy burdens from the past into the future makes it difficult for us to fully enjoy life.

A Stanford University study found college students trained to forgive someone who had hurt them were significantly less angry, more hopeful and better able to deal with emotions than students not trained to forgive.[3] A survey of 1,400 adults found that having the willingness to forgive oneself and others, and the feeling of being forgiven, have beneficial health effects.[4] Researchers have found that anger and resentment cause stress hormones to accumulate in the blood and that forgiveness reduces this buildup.

When we hold onto hurt, we hand control of our emotions to another person. In doing so, it does not change them, but it changes us and steals our sense of peace and joy. When we are unforgiving, bitterness seeps into our entire being, impairing all our attitudes and relationships, creating anger, jealousy, resentment, hatred and envy in us. Unforgiveness causes division, wounding and brokenness in relationships. It becomes a barrier to creating healthy relationships for fear we will be hurt again.

Refusing to forgive may be likened to drinking poison and hoping it kills the other person. When we forgive, we extend love and mercy to someone who has wronged or hurt us, releasing the hostility and resentment from our hurts. It is not something we arrive at easily, nor is it something we do out of fear or obligation or to keep peace within relationships. It is something we do for ourselves.

Forgiveness doesn't mean we forget the hurt or continue to accept repeated mistreatment, but it is an action we take to free ourselves

3. Frederick M. Luskin, Kenneth Ginzburg, and Christopher E. Thoresen, "The Effect of Forgiveness Training on Psychosocial Factors in College-Age Adults," in "Altruism, Intergroup Apology and Forgiveness: Antidote for a Divided World," special issue, *Humboldt Journal of Social Relations* 29, no. 2 (2005): 163–184.

4. Loren L. Toussaint et al., "Forgiveness and Health: Age Differences in a U.S. Probability Sample," *Journal of Adult Development* 8 (2001): 249–257.

from the burden and pain we carry. When we forgive others, space is created in our lives to heal and grow as we move beyond the offense to create peace about it instead of anger or bitterness. We can forgive and rebuild damaged relationships, or we can forgive and still choose to distance ourselves from the people who have hurt and mistreated us or continue to hurt and mistreat us.

> *"We can't hold a man down without staying down with him."*
> — Booker T. Washington (1856–1915), American educator, author and political leader

Forgiveness is not only about forgiving the person. It also requires us to set aside the remembrance of the offense, except to establish appropriate boundaries, and not to bring it up again in anger or spite. Forgiveness is a process where we learn to detach from the hurt and anxiety and set ourselves free. It changes lives and reminds us that we are equal with every other person. We all do good and noble things and we all offend others.

One of the most forgiving acts we can do is not to judge. When we are self-righteous, we separate ourselves from others and may engage in hateful and negative thoughts toward them. This attitude keeps us trapped.

Hurt people hurt people, so having empathy and compassion for someone else's life struggles and mistakes makes it easier to forgive them. Instead of dwelling on people's thoughtless words or behaviors, we can make a habit of forgiving them. Doing so prevents us from holding onto the offence as we let go of the past and move on to a brighter and more productive future.

The process of forgiving also includes forgiving ourselves for past mistakes, foibles and failures. Learning to forgive ourselves comes from offering compassion and understanding toward ourselves. Doing so clears the way to reconcile and strengthen relationships in our lives.

Consider some of the following components of forgiveness as you practice it:

- Forgiveness never keeps score.
- Forgiveness never boasts of its own record.
- Forgiveness never complains.
- Forgiveness does not have a martyr syndrome.
- Forgiveness is not envious, jealous or angry when another does well.
- Forgiveness does not alienate, divide or separate.

Embracing Health, Balance and Abundance with Your Family

Supportive family relationships enhance your life and your health. You cannot choose the family you are born into, but you can choose how you interact and show your **LOVE** for them. Doing so requires **L**istening, **O**verlooking, **V**alidating and **E**ffort. It is not something to be left to chance.

It takes couples who are honest, committed and supportive toward each other. It takes parents' being involved in their children's lives. It takes learning better ways to define and communicate your boundaries, discipline your choice of words and offer forgiveness. It may even involve addressing the issues of addiction or abuse.

It takes **GUTS** to build a loving, caring and supportive family unit. There will be times when you need to **G**et **U**ncomfortable **T**o **S**ucceed, but know you can do it by saying and challenging yourself to …

Let It Begin with Me!

Chapter 5

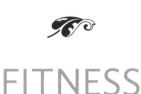

FITNESS

How Do You Treat Your Body, Mind and Soul?

Star athletes, award-winning musicians and top-earning executives become good at what they do only with persistent work and vigilance. They discipline themselves mentally and physically. They practice regularly to build their physical and mental stamina. Their bodies need to function in harmony, integrally and in balance every day as they know their physical and mental health affect everything they do. When we develop habits of good nutrition, daily activity and positive thinking, we are more successful and have improved health and enjoyment in life.

> *"Take good care of your body. It's the only place you have to live."*
>
> — Jim Rohn (1930–2009), American entrepreneur, author and motivational speaker

Not everyone can be at the top, but we can all strive to be better. Without healthy bodies, minds and souls, we limit what we can do and accomplish in life. When we take proper care of our bodies, we will have a comfortable place in which to live for many years. But we can't buy new bodies, improved health or our lives back after years of neglect.

Taking care of your body includes physical and nutritional fitness as well as environmental, mental, emotional and spiritual fitness. These six components work together to keep your body functioning in harmony, while enhancing your endurance, strength and flexibility to maintain all the other parts of your balance wheel of health and well-being. This chapter highlights these six components of fitness; explains the benefits of maintaining them to optimize your body, mind and soul; and provides **TIP**s and **ABC**s to help you improve each of them.

> *"If you can hold the progress of disease in check, and if you can stimulate and enhance [your] own defense mechanisms (which is your immune system), there are no diseases which your body is not capable of conquering."*
>
> — Terry Pulse, American physician

> *"Your lifestyle— how you live, eat, emote, and think— determines your health. To prevent disease, you may have to change how you live."*
>
> — Brian Carter, American author and speaker

Physical Fitness

The human body is designed for activity. Years ago we were a society of hunters and gatherers. Our survival depended on our bodies' ability to be flexible and strong. Today, many of us scarcely move, spending our days in sedentary jobs and then driving home for an evening of television, surfing the Internet or playing video games. This inactivity is as bad for us as a diet of bread and bacon.

When a car idles too long, its engine stalls. When we lead sedentary lives, it's like putting the brakes on our metabolism. Just walking slowly burns three calories per minute, whereas sitting burns only one calorie per minute. When we are idle, our triglyceride and blood sugar levels rise. Inactivity lowers our good cholesterol (HDL) and puts us at risk of weight gain, diabetes, heart disease and a variety of cancers.

Modern entertainment and labor-saving devices, from cars to computers to elevators, create disastrous effects on our physical health, not to mention our waistlines. Surveys find that a quarter of our population never engage in physical activity, and sixty percent don't engage in enough to keep fit.

When our bodies are physically fit, our body systems function at their best, aiding in the prevention of disease, boosting energy, reducing stress and benefiting our emotional well-being. To combat disease and premature aging, our bones, joints and muscles must be flexible and strong. A complete physical fitness routine incorporates a combination of endurance, strength and flexibility exercises. Finding time and ways to balance a combination of all three while having fun is the ultimate goal.

> *"Make rest a necessity not an objective. Only rest long enough to gather strength."*
>
> — Jim Rohn (1930–2009), American entrepreneur, author and motivational speaker

Endurance exercises get the large muscles of our bodies working; they make our hearts beat faster and our lungs work harder. Activities such as walking, jogging, cycling and swimming help build endurance.

Strengthening exercises involve working our muscles against resistance. Lifting weights is good for building and maintaining muscle strength, but using a pair of cans from the kitchen cupboard also works. Strengthening exercises make it easier to perform daily activities such as carrying the groceries, doing yard work or shoveling snow. As we become older, strengthening exercises make a huge difference in our ability to climb stairs and get out of an easy chair.

Flexibility exercises help keep our bodies limber, making it easier for us to move about. I remember my kindergarten teacher encouraging her young students to stay flexible by singing "bend and stretch, reach for the sky, stand on tippy toes, oh so high!" Stretching and reaching helps increase our range of motion, giving us the ability to walk, golf, ski and garden, and even tie our shoes more easily.

In his book *Living the Good Life: Your Guide to Health and Success*, David Patchell-Evans, president and CEO of GoodLife Fitness clubs, comments that people often say they don't have time to exercise. However, studies show we are, at a minimum, twenty percent more productive when we exercise. There are only 168 hours in a week, but by exercising we gain more time. We are able to make decisions twenty percent faster and have twenty percent less anxiety and twenty percent deeper sleep. When we exercise for half an hour three times a week, that hour and a half a week translates into added hours of productive time and another two or more years of life. Not a bad deal! Without a physical fitness routine in our lives, we actually lose time.

A reader of *Younger Next Year: Live Strong, Fit, and Sexy—Until You're 80 and Beyond* by Chris Crowley and Dr. Henry Lodge called the book "a twenty-first century fountain of youth." Dr. Lodge writes, "Some 70 percent of premature death and aging is lifestyle-related." He found the more he looked at the science of aging, the more it became clear that many of our ailments are *not* a normal part of growing old. He argues that many illnesses, such as heart attacks, strokes, the common cancers, diabetes, most falls, fractures and serious injuries, are primarily caused by the way we live. He says, "If we had the will to do it, we could eliminate more than half of all disease in women and men over fifty. Not delay it, eliminate it!"

Many of us may well live into our nineties, whether we like it or not. How we live those years is largely under our control. In expressing why he wrote *Younger Next Year*, Dr. Lodge stated, "I cannot, as a doctor, sit here and watch people I care for and care about go down a road that is leading them to an awful place without doing something. It is not enough to wait for the car to crash and then do a good job of treating the injured and dying. If 70 percent of the serious illness I see is preventable, then it's my job to prevent it."

Our bodies and brains are perfect for their natural purposes, but they are not designed for a life that includes fast food, TV and idleness. Our bodies are designed for life in nature, where the fit survive. Dr. Lodge uses the analogy: "Most of your body parts have as little business in a mall as a saber-tooth tiger." He goes on to say that aging is inevitable, but some of what we dread about aging, and what we call aging, is actually decay. Biologically, when we age our hair turns gray, our heart rate declines, our skin degenerates and so on, so we *look* old, but we do not have to *act* or *feel* old.

As we age, especially as we head into our forties and fifties, our bodies begin to trigger the "default to decay" setting, where it stops sending out signals to grow and begins to age instead. At this time, we can "override those default signals, swim against the tide and change decay back into growth." Dr. Lodge reiterates, the keys to supersede the decay of our bodies are daily exercise, nutrition, emotional stability and being engaged in living our lives, but it begins with exercise.

The best six doctors anywhere
And no one can deny it
Are sunshine, water, rest, and air
Exercise and diet.
These six will gladly you attend
If only you are willing
Your mind they'll ease
Your will they'll mend
And charge you not a shilling.

— **Nursery rhyme**

When we exercise, our bodies send out chemical signals to help us become lean, powerful and efficient. Exercise reverses the chemistry of decay. When we exercise regularly,

- we lose excess fat;

- our bone strength and joint health increase;

- our heart and circulation functions increase to deliver oxygen and nourishment to our muscles;

- our muscles become strong, supple and more coordinated;

- our immune functions increase to repair the ongoing wear and tear from sprains, cuts, bruises and minor infections that accompany active living;

- our brains develop a chemistry of optimism, leading to increased curiosity and a willingness to explore new things and interact more with others, as well as increased energy and alertness; and

- our mortality rates decrease.

"In minds crammed with thoughts, organs clogged with toxins and bodies stiffened with neglect, there is just no space for anything else."

— Alison Rose Levy, American health journalist

In my understanding of the economics of health, these results are phenomenal. Investing in exercise offers us large dividends. Remaining active by investing in regular exercise offers us a bountiful **R**eturn **O**n **L**ife, or **ROL**.

David Patchell-Evans also highlights numerous other ways exercise gives us a positive **ROL**, stating that exercise

- increases our self-confidence and self-esteem;

- improves our digestion and appetite for healthful food;

- helps us sleep better;

- gives us more energy, endurance and strength;

- improves our body shape;

- burns extra calories, increasing the enzymes that burn fat;

- tones and firms our muscles;

- improves circulation and helps lower blood pressure;
- lifts our spirits, reducing tension and stress;
- strengthens the heart, improving blood flow through the body;
- enhances the function of the respiratory system;
- improves bone metabolism, decreasing the chances of developing osteoporosis;
- improves the development and strength of connective tissue;
- lowers the risk of death from cancer;
- improves resistance to infectious disease;
- enhances clarity of mind, improving our emotional stability and alleviating depression;
- alleviates constipation;
- enables us to meet new friends and develop fulfilling relationships;
- helps us move past self-imposed limitations;
- gives us a greater appreciation for life;
- enables us to enjoy all types of physical activities;
- makes our clothes look better on us;
- improves athletic performance and enhances sexual performance;
- reduces joint discomfort, increasing range of motion;
- gets our minds off irritations, reducing and preventing boredom;
- gives us a clearer perspective on ideas, issues, problems and challenges;
- affords us the opportunity to experience our potential, giving us a greater desire to participate in life; and
- helps us live longer.

The key to being physically fit is to stay active. But many find it challenging to go to the gym regularly or to fit more activity into their busy days. A concept called NEAT (non-exercise activity thermogenesis) can help. Proposed by Dr. James Levine at the Mayo Clinic, this concept shows that if we do brief, low-intensity physical activity regularly, we can burn from 300 to 1,000 calories a day and offset the danger from all the sitting we cannot avoid.

A Better **C**hoice and some "neat" ways to help you keep moving include

- walking to work or getting off the bus or train a stop early and walking the rest of the way;
- taking the stairs;
- parking at the far end of the parking lot, whether at the shopping mall or the office;
- programming regular breaks into your workday and walking around your office while visiting your colleagues in person rather than calling or emailing them;
- walking or riding your bike to the neighborhood store;
- going for a twenty-minute walk at lunchtime;
- standing whenever possible, such as when you are on the phone;
- when you have extra time before an appointment, walking up and down the hall or doing some calf or leg raises;
- keeping comfortable shoes close by to use whenever an opportunity to exercise arises;
- recruiting an activity buddy (you are more likely to persevere when you have someone else to encourage you and keep you accountable);
- washing the car, working in the garden, cleaning out a closet or dancing;

- doing sit-ups, jumping on a trampoline, riding a stationary bike or walking on the treadmill while watching TV;

- hiding the TV remote and getting up to change the channel or turn off the TV; and

- playing with your children, going for a walk or playing fetch with your dog.

> *"A man's health can be judged by which he takes two at a time—pills or stairs."*
> — Joan Welsh, American author

LOOK GOOD, FEEL GOOD

Being physically fit also includes our personal appearance. Proper grooming and healthful personal habits ward off illness and help us feel good about ourselves, make us more attractive, help us present a professional appearance and provide mental benefits.

Donald Novey, a physician with the Advocate Medical Group in Park Ridge, Illinois, encourages the practice of good body hygiene as a way to help us feel good about ourselves and improve our mental health. He says people with poor hygiene habits, unkempt hair and clothes, body odor, bad breath, missing teeth and the like are often seen as unhealthy. Because of this, they may face discrimination and depression.

Here are some of Dr. Novey's personal care **TIP**s:

- Bathe regularly: Washing at regular intervals sheds dead skin and odor.

- Take care of your hair and scalp: Washing and conditioning hair improves its texture and appearance and reduces or eliminates dandruff.

- Trim your nails: Trimming fingernails and toenails keeps them in good shape and helps prevent hangnails and infected nail beds. It also provides an opportunity to inspect your feet for other problems.

- Brush and floss your teeth: Brushing and flossing minimizes tooth decay, gum disease and bad breath by decreasing the accumulation of bacteria in your mouth. Six-month dental visits help maintain a healthy smile.

- Wash your hands: Washing hands before preparing or eating food and after using the bathroom, coughing or sneezing and handling garbage prevents the spread of bacteria and viruses.

- Sleep tight: Seven to ten hours of sleep a night refreshes you and allows your body to repair itself while boosting the immune system.

- Treat your clothing with care: Keeping clothes in good repair, ensuring everything matches, and dressing appropriately for the occasion gives you a neat and clean appearance.

- Care for your health: Yearly or bi-yearly medical checkups promote good health and facilitate early detection of serious problems.

SMILE AND THE WHOLE WORLD SMILES WITH YOU!

When we are pleasant and cheerful, we put other people at ease, but when we're sour or unpleasant, everyone around us feels uncomfortable and insecure. When we relax and smile, we feel better, and so do others—it makes everyone feel confident. Smiling decreases stress and makes us look better and more attractive. It's a simple, low-energy and cost-efficient way to help us feel better.

According to plastic surgeon Dr. David Song, assistant professor at the University of Chicago Hospitals, it takes eight muscles to smile and nine to frown. He explains that when we smile genuinely, it takes two muscles to crinkle our eyes, two to pull up our lip corners and nose, two to elevate the mouth angle and two to pull the mouth corners sideways. When we frown, we use two to pull down our lips and wrinkle our lower face, three to crease our brow, one to purse our lips, one to depress our lower lip and two to pull the corners of our mouth down. He also says a fake smile uses only two muscles and can be detected because the eyes don't smile.

Ten reasons to make smiling **A B**etter **C**hoice:

1. Smiling makes you attractive: We're drawn to people who smile; it's an attraction factor. Frowns, scowls and grimaces push people away.

2. Smiling changes your mood: Smiling tricks your body into changing your mood for the better.

3. Smiling is contagious: Smiling lightens up a room and changes the moods of others, making everyone happier.

4. Smiling relieves stress: Smiling helps prevent you from feeling tired, worn down, overwhelmed and stressed, making you better able to take action.

5. Smiling boosts your immune system: Smiling relaxes you, which helps your immune system function better.

6. Smiling lowers your blood pressure: When you are relaxed your blood pressure stabilizes.

7. Smiling releases endorphins, natural painkillers and serotonin: Smiling is a natural drug, causing you to feel good.

8. Smiling lifts the face and makes you look younger: The muscles you use to smile lift your face.

9. Smiling makes you seem successful: Smiling people appear more confident and are more likely to be promoted and approached. When you smile at meetings and appointments, people react to you differently.

10. Smiling helps you stay positive: Try this test: Smile. Now try to think of something negative without losing the smile. It's hard. When you smile, your body sends you a message that life is good!

Nutritional Fitness

What we eat and drink provides energy for our bodies' growth, maintenance and repair, and for physical and mental activity. Our bodies are like high-powered, finely engineered vehicles, but instead of being powered by gasoline, they are powered by the food we eat. What we put into our fuel tanks is burned by our activity; however, low-octane fuel—or junk food—clogs up our bodies—or our engines. Eating healthful food keeps our bodies functioning at a higher level.

> **"You are what you eat!"**
> — Victor Hugo Lindlahr, (1897–1969), American health food and weight-loss pioneer

Just like finely engineered vehicles, our bodies speak to us when something is wrong. We may notice problems only once our bodies are not operating well or are completely damaged. But unlike vehicles, acquiring spare parts for our bodies is not a viable option.

Healthful food choices help control cholesterol, diabetes, obesity and high blood pressure. They help us maintain a healthy weight, prevent heart disease and cancer and have a major impact on degenerative diseases. Healthful foods give us more energy and stabilize us emotionally and mentally so we can perform at optimal levels.

> **"He who takes medicine and neglects to diet wastes the skill of his doctors."**
> — Chinese proverb

Often, the more convenient the food, the less healthful it is. A diet low in fats with sufficient protein and high in fiber, fruits and vegetables protects us against disease. Junk and processed foods, which are low in fiber and high in fats, sugar and chemical additives, do not protect us. Unhealthful foods affect the way we feel, think and respond to life's challenges.

Following are nutritional **TIP**s **T**o **I**mprove your **P**erformance in avoiding the effects of the **M**odern **A**merican **D**iet, or **MAD**:

- Eat a low-fat diet, keeping fat intake to fifteen percent of daily calories. Eat lots of fresh fruits and vegetables, use low-fat dressings and cheese, eat lean meats that are baked or broiled and use nonhydrogenated oils.

- Eat forty to fifty grams of mixed fibers daily to protect against colon cancer, lower cholesterol and stabilize blood sugar. There are two types of fiber:

    i. Soluble fiber, which controls blood sugar and lowers blood cholesterol. It is found in oat bran, oatmeal, beans, peas and lentils.

    ii. Insoluble fiber, known as roughage, which prevents and controls bowel problems. It is found in wheat bran, rye bread, brown rice and fresh fruits and vegetables.

- Eat a low-salt diet to reduce fluid retention, decreasing the need for your heart to work hard.

- Eat fresh or fresh frozen vegetables instead of canned or bottled ones.

- Avoid processed foods such as deli meats, dry soup mixes, casserole mixes, salted nuts and chips.

- Use fresh or dried herbs and spices, lemon juice and flavored vinegars.

- Eat a low-sugar or no-sugar diet.

ACID VERSUS ALKALINE

A healthful, well-balanced diet creates a proper acid/alkaline, or pH, balance in our bodies. It helps maintain our internal equilibrium, or homeostasis. Science has discovered that disease organisms prefer an acidic rather than an alkaline environment.

Picture a swamp—thick, wet, sticky, humid, muddy, creepy and full of bugs. Now picture a lush meadow that is pleasing to your senses—rich dark loam, colorful flowers, rabbits running through it and beautiful butterflies fluttering about. The sun is shining and the air is clear as sunflowers and wild honeysuckle blow in the warm, gentle breeze.

An acidic body is like the swamp, attracting illness and disease and causing discomfort. An alkaline body is like the meadow, where peace, contentment and good health abound. Which environment would you prefer to live in?

Many people's body chemistry is acidic due to our **MAD** diet and lifestyle choices. The millions of dollars spent on antacids is proof of this. Calcium is used by our bodies as a buffering agent to alkalize high acidity. If there is not enough calcium in our diet, it is pulled from our bones and teeth. Left unchecked, this process has a negative effect on our bone density and dental health.

Many books on nutrition discuss alkaline and acidic foods. The authors of these books may list foods in different categories, depending on the research criteria used. My list is based on the work of Dr. Elson M. Haas in his book *Staying Healthy with Nutrition: The Complete Guide to Diet and Nutritional Medicine*, which was recommended to me by a nutritionist friend who calls it the "nutrition bible." Dr. Haas lists alkaline- and acid-forming foods, as well as foods that balance alkalinity and acidity.

- Alkaline-forming foods: All vegetables, most fruits, millet, buckwheat, sprouted beans, olive oil and soaked almonds

- Acid-forming foods: Wheat, oats, white rice, pomegranates, strawberries, breads, refined flour, refined sugar, cashews, pecans, peanuts, butter, cheese, eggs, meat, fish and poultry

- Balancing foods: Brown rice, corn, soybeans, lima beans, almonds, sunflower seeds, Brazil nuts, honey, most dried beans and peas, tofu, nonfat milk and vegetable oils other than olive oil

Tobacco, chemical pollutants, toxins, prescription drugs, over-the-counter drugs and illegal drugs, combined with stress and emotional upset, also cause our bodies to become more acidic, creating an internal swamp-like condition and opening the door for illness and disease to set in.

VITAMIN AND MINERAL SUPPLEMENTS

We are exposed to many chemicals, pesticides and pollutants that seep into the water we drink. They are absorbed into the food we eat and permeate the air we breathe. A study analyzing the blood of newborns in the United States found their blood contained seventy-six chemicals that damage cells in humans and animals, ninety-four that are toxic to the brain and nervous system and seventy-nine that are toxic to a developing fetus.[1]

Various studies show how overfarming, the use of chemical fertilizers, soil contamination and soil erosion result in the depletion of minerals and other nutrients in our fruits and vegetables. A recent report by the United States Department of Agriculture showed the following amounts of vitamins and minerals have been lost in fruits and vegetables since 1975:

- Apples: Vitamin A is down forty-one percent.
- Sweet peppers: Vitamin C is down thirty-one percent.
- Watercress: Iron is down eighty-eight percent.
- Broccoli: Calcium and vitamin A are each down fifty percent.
- Cauliflower: Vitamin C is down forty-five percent, vitamin B1 is down forty-eight percent and vitamin B2 is down forty-seven percent.

---

1. Environmental Working Group, "Pollution in People: Cord Blood Contaminants in Minority Newborns," Environmental Working Group Publication (2009), www.ewg.org/files/2009-Minority-Cord-Blood-Report.pdf.

• Collard greens: Magnesium is down eighty-five percent.[2]

A Better **C**hoice to help us sustain good health would be to consider a daily regimen of vitamin and mineral supplements. Taking daily supplements is a great way to ensure you are getting all the nutrients you need to stay healthy.

The word *supplement* means "something added." Be careful when adding supplements if you are prescribed drugs or therapy for a medical condition or disease. Some supplements are contraindicated with certain prescription drugs.

Also be aware that an herbal supplement or a vitamin regimen won't cure your health problem, and not all supplements are good, especially when taken in large doses.

Media and advertising often mislead us by promising "totally safe," "natural" or "quick and effective" solutions to health problems. Keep yourself safe by researching any product you consider taking. Ensure there is valid scientific research supporting the claims of marketers.

READING LABELS

Reading labels on food products provides a snapshot of what the food contains. To increase your understanding of food labels here are some **TIP**s:

• Ingredients are listed in the order of their volume, the largest amount listed first and the least listed last.

• Energy is expressed as the number of calories per serving.

• Nutritional content is given per serving.

• Salt can be listed as salt, MSG, sodium, baking soda, baking powder, brine, soy sauce or spices.

---

2. "Vegetables without Vitamins," *Life Extension Magazine* (March 2001), www.lef.
org/magazine/mag2001/mar2001_report_vegetables.html.

- Sugars are listed as sugar, honey, molasses and anything ending in *ose*—dextrose, sucrose, fructose, maltose and lactose—as well as dextrin, maltodextrin or syrups.

- Fats can be listed as fat, lard, shortening, oils, monoglycerides, triglycerides or tallow.

A Better **C**hoice when purchasing foods is to consider choosing items with five or fewer ingredients and staying away from those with words on the label that you cannot pronounce.

EATING OUT

Eating out is fun and convenient but, depending on the restaurants chosen and how frequently you eat out, you can do yourself, your children and your grandchildren a dangerous, long-term disservice. Eating at fast-food restaurants and from drive-through establishments usually results in eating high-fat, nutritionally deficient meals.

Choose wisely when you eat out. Find restaurants offering low-fat alternatives. Order broiled or baked foods, not fried. Choose milk for coffee instead of cream, dressing on the side so you can use only a little and plain rice or a baked potato instead of french fries. Try stir-fries with lots of vegetables. For dessert choose fresh fruit, sherbet, frozen yogurt or a specialty coffee. Aim to stay away from the **MAD** foods.

WATER

Water is one of the most important elements of our bodies. It makes up approximately seventy percent of our muscles and seventy-five percent of our brains. Water plays a vital role in the proper functioning of our bodies and is an essential part of a healthful diet.

Water suppresses the appetite, aids in digestion, helps circulate nutrients and oxygen through the body and assists the body in eliminating waste. Water lubricates joints, protects organs, helps maintain normal body temperature and is necessary for exercise and day-to-day performance. It gives us healthier skin, hair and nails and increases energy and alertness.

It has been suggested that water is the single most important ingredient in determining diet and fitness success as it forces fat to be used as fuel. Without adequate water, our kidneys cannot function properly. This prompts the liver to pick up the slack, causing additional problems as the liver can't properly metabolize stored fat, resulting in more fat being stored in the body.

The suggested minimum daily serving of water is six eight-ounce glasses. **TIP**s for reaching your water intake include the following:

- Drink a glass of water between every meal and a glass in the evening.
- Take a bottle of water wherever you go. Sip on it all day.
- Reach for water instead of high-sugar, high-fat snacks.

Here are some interesting facts about water:

- One glass of water shuts down hunger pangs.
- Lack of water is the number one trigger of daytime fatigue.
- Research indicates that eight to ten glasses of water a day significantly eases back and joint pain.
- A two percent drop in body water can trigger fuzzy short-term memory, trouble with basic math and difficulty focusing on the computer screen.
- Drinking six glasses of water daily decreases the risk of colon cancer by forty-five percent and breast cancer by seventy-nine percent and makes us fifty percent less likely to develop bladder cancer.

OTHER NUTRITIONAL TIPS

Your physical, mental and emotional fitness is enhanced when you eat well. You feel better, think better, work more effectively and have more fun.

Good eating habits take practice to become second nature. Pick one or two of the following healthful eating **TIP**s and commit to making them work in your life, then pick another as you continue to improve your eating habits.

- Eat when you're hungry; aim for six smaller meals per day.
- Eat a variety of foods for balanced nutrition.
- Enjoy what you eat; spice foods up for different flavors.
- Eat sitting down; people eat more while standing up.
- Put down your fork and knife or spoon between each bite.
- Eat from a smaller plate.
- Eat slowly; after twenty minutes of eating, our brains send a message that we are full.
- Stop eating when you are no longer hungry.
- Eat smaller portions more frequently rather than one or two large meals.
- Keep high-calorie, high-fat and low-quality foods out of your fridge, pantry and home.
- Stay focused on things you need to do and keep your mind off food; ask yourself if you really need something before mindlessly putting it in your mouth.
- Be aware of your emotions when you eat.

Environmental Fitness

What does the environment you live and work in look, sound and smell like? How do you feel when you are in these environments? The physical condition—the sights, sounds and smells—of our homes, workplaces and where we spend our time impact our overall fitness and health.

Just as it's important to take care of our bodies internally and externally, it's important to take care of the spaces in which we live, work and play. Clutter and dirt open the door for germs and bacteria to grow, leading to illness and disease. They create unpleasant and uncomfortable environments in which to live.

The sound of constant and/or loud noises leads to cluttered and unhealthy minds, as well as hearing damage. Soothing sounds and silence can calm our thoughts and promote more creative thinking and peaceful minds.

Smells can nauseate us or help us feel relaxed and energized. Did you know our bodies can distinguish around 10,000 different scents? When we inhale, scents travel across the olfactory nerves located inside the nose and into the part of the brain that controls our moods, memory and ability to learn. This area is called the *limbic system*, and when stimulated it releases endorphins, neurotransmitters and other "feel-good" chemicals. Good smells can boost our immune, respiratory and circulatory systems, while offering us relaxation and stress relief, mood enhancement and well-being.

On the other hand, products used to clean and add aroma to our environments may trigger serious reactions for some, leading to illness, absence from work and even hospitalization. These chemicals vaporize and are easily inhaled, causing respiratory irritations and breathing difficulties. Some cause skin reactions and others can trigger vascular changes that may lead to asthma or migraine headaches. People who are susceptible can experience symptoms, even from very low levels of chemicals.

Most people spend eighty to ninety percent of their time indoors. It is in these environments that we are most likely to be exposed to chemicals that are toxic. They create poor indoor air quality, which exacerbates allergies and asthma; they cause eye, nose and throat irritation, along with fatigue, nausea and illness. Carpets, humidity, pesticides, biological pollutants, asbestos, radon, mold and carbon monoxide all cause air-quality problems. Exposure to chemicals in mouthwash, hair conditioner, cologne or perfume, laundry detergent, window cleaner and more can create a chemical soup in our bodies, which, after long-term exposure, can lead to illness and disease.

Environment Protection Agency studies find that even in urban areas with high levels of industrial pollution, the concentration of toxic chemicals is higher indoors than outdoors, in some cases up to seventy times higher. These chemicals can enter our bodies from the food and drink we consume, by breathing it in and by absorbing it through our skin.

Keeping the environments in which you live, work and play healthy by maintaining cleanliness and tidiness, listening to sounds that are calming and peaceful and eliminating the use of toxic chemicals and fragrances will increase physical and mental health and boost energy levels.

Mental Fitness

Remember the high-powered, finely engineered vehicle I mentioned in the discussion on nutritional fitness? Well, imagine your mind as the driver of that vehicle taking control and either steering your body to victory or causing you to hit the wall. Just as the shape and condition of your body is determined by the food you feed it and the exercise you give it, so is the condition of your mind determined by what you feed it and the exercise you give it. And just as the finely engineered vehicle needs an oil change, you may need a change in the way you nurture your mind.

"Intellectual growth should commence at birth and cease only at death."

— Albert Einstein (1879–1955), German theoretical physicist

The average adult thinks 60,000 thoughts per day. What type of thoughts flow through your mind? What do you say to yourself?

We communicate to ourselves through our minds with words and pictures. Every waking moment, we mold our self-image with the thoughts and images we create of ourselves and our daily performance. This affects our self-esteem, attitudes and moods.

Watch your thoughts, for they become words.
Watch your words, for they become actions.
Watch your actions, for they become habits.
Watch your habits, for they become character.
Watch your character, for it becomes your destiny.

— Author unknown

It is important to be mindful of your mental thoughts and images. It's important to spend time examining your thought life. Ask yourself, "What am I thinking about?" "What am I saying to myself?" Actively become aware of your thoughts and their patterns. Many of us tend to relate unhappiness with what is going on around us or to our circumstances, but unhappiness is often related to what is going on in our minds with our personal thoughts and inner conversations.

We can control the language of our minds to work for us, and as a result, our self-confidence and outlook on life improve. Allowing only positive and affirming thoughts to dwell in our minds takes awareness and practice. Saying, "That's more like it," "Things are working out well" or "I'll do it better next time" are good for our mental health and self-esteem; it is like having a nurturing coach with us all the time.

> *"Thought is creative. You create your entire life with your thoughts, hour by hour and minute by minute."*
> — Brian Tracy, Canadian author and motivational speaker

You may not always have control over what pops into your head, but you do have control over what stays there. You can send the negative thoughts away and keep the positive ones. Imagine your brain as having the same functions as a computer—activate the "delete" function and dissolve negative thoughts. Then activate positive thoughts to fill your mind with new possibilities and improved outcomes.

A study by Rutgers University sociologist Ellen Idler and epidemiologist Stanislov Kasl of Yale University School of Medicine found that the thoughts we think and the words we say affect our physical health and well-being. In their study of 2,800 men and women over sixty-five years of age, they found a person's answer to the question, "Is your health excellent, good, fair or poor?" is a predictor of who will live or die in the next four years. According to their findings, which were corroborated by five other large studies totaling 23,000 people, those who rated their health as poor were four to five times more likely to die in that time than those who rated their health as excellent. These findings remained true, even for the individuals who rated their health as poor but were actually in comparable health to those who rated their health as excellent.[3]

> "The game of life is the game of boomerangs. Our thoughts, deeds and words return to us sooner or later, with astounding accuracy."
> — Florence Shinn (1871–1940), American artist, book illustrator and author

Our thoughts chart a course for us. They point us in the direction in which our lives will go. They cause us to have certain attitudes and perspectives that affect our relationships, determine our productivity and influence the quality of our lives.

In 1997, my thoughts were very negative. After meeting with my doctor and telling her, "I don't like myself anymore!" she sent me to a psychiatrist. He gave me a diagnosis of major depression and anxiety. I received counseling and medication. In time, my condition improved and I have not required counseling or medication for many years. Since my bout with mental illness, I have become more and

---

3. Ellen L. Idler and Stanislav Kasl, "Health Perceptions and Survival: Do Global Evaluations of Health Status Really Predict Mortality?" *Journal of Gerontology* 46, no. 2 (1991): S55–65.

more aware of my thoughts and how different stimuli and situations affect my mental health and well-being.

My mind can become a battlefield of conflicting thoughts, where my negative or "stinking thinking" brings my day to a crawl, putting me into the pit of despair and pulling me down. When negative thinking begins to attack my mind, my day spirals downward. It is not until I become aware of these thoughts and consciously refuse to let them continue to bombard my mind that the outcome of my day changes.

> *"The life you are leading is simply a reflection of your thinking."*
>
> — Doug Firebaugh, American trainer, speaker and author

When I refuse to allow negative thoughts to take hold of me and lead me, I am able to turn my day around to be one that is enjoyable and productive.

It has taken a great deal of practice and diligence to become proficient at sending my unhealthful, negative thoughts away. More often than not, the only way I can sustain a peaceful and positive mind is by concentrating on and saying words that create affirmative thoughts, feelings and actions. Destructive thoughts bring me failure, whereas good thoughts dramatically increase my chances for success.

Saying positive affirmations such as "I am loved, I am accepted, I am confident and all is well" leads to better outcomes. A friend of mine uses "Always free, always safe, always secure" as a positive affirmation when she is struggling with negative thoughts.

> *"Garbage in, garbage out!"*
>
> — George Fuechsel, American computer technician

We are what we think we are! There was a woman who had a persistent fever, but her doctors couldn't find anything physically wrong. They questioned her thoroughly and discovered when she became upset about anything, she would always say, "That just burns me up." She used the phrase several times a day. Her doctors weren't sure if it had anything to do with her condition, but they asked her not to use the phrase anymore. Within weeks her body temperature returned to normal.

How many times have we heard people say, "Every time I eat that, it makes me sick," "My back is just killing me" or "Those kids make me nervous." Our own words give instructions to our bodies and to our immune systems. Our bodies will eventually respond to our instructions.

What we listen to, read and see affect what we think and say, and what we think and say impacts our mental health. Did you know that the average person is exposed to nine hours of media every day? Think about the information that is shared and received through various media. How does this information affect the way you think, feel and act?

Become aware of the mental nutrition you feed your mind. Reevaluate how good and how healthful this diet is to your mental health. To help you analyze the impact of what you hear, see and read, consider your answers to the following questions:

- What are the lyrics of the songs I listen to?
- What type of TV programs do I watch? How long and how often do I watch them? What do the characters say to each other?
- When I surf the Internet, what types of sites do I go to?
- Do I go to bed with the eleven o'clock news and wake up to the morning news?
- What types of books do I read?
- Do I take courses to improve my skills and increase my knowledge?

An essential component of mental fitness is to keep our brains active and stimulated. Our brains are the control centers of our bodies. They are the storehouses for our memories and where all learning

"I'm still learning."

— Michelangelo (1475–1564), Italian Renaissance sculptor, painter, architect and poet

begins. They are our center of reason. Keeping our brains active through lifelong learning improves our mental health. Taking courses and learning new skills keeps our minds and brains active and keeps us growing. By continuing to learn we can balance and enhance the skills and knowledge we have already mastered. It helps us stay and feel younger and more vibrant.

Another way to improve mental health and well-being is through gratitude. It has been shown that people who keep a gratitude journal, in which they write things they are grateful for, are more likely to exercise regularly, experience fewer physical symptoms, be more optimistic about the future and be more likely to attain their personal, academic, interpersonal and health-related goals. They feel better.

Consider the **B**lessings, **A**ccomplishments and **G**oals you're thankful for daily. Your gratitude meter will grow dramatically when you open your **BAG** of life regularly to count up what's there.

- **B**lessings, or what you're endowed with: Life, health and living in a free and abundant country; your family, friends and work; the air you breathe, clothes you wear and food you eat. For a challenge and some fun, name your **B**lessings starting with A and going to Z.

- **A**ccomplishments, or what you have learned and accomplished in life: Learned to walk, talk and ride a bike; finished high school, college or university; or completed a special project at home or at work. In listing your accomplishments, don't compare yourself with others, because *to compare is to despair.*

- **G**oals, or your plans, hopes and dreams: The special trip with your family, the car you desire or the house you want to call home. They are motivators.

Your **BAG** of life, along with the following **TIP**s, will enhance and improve your mental fitness:

- Accept that you alone can control your thoughts; ensure what you say and think are positive and affirming.

- Evaluate what you feed your mind—what you read, see and hear. Ask yourself, "Is this going to help my personal, family and work life?" "Will it build me up or tear me down?"

- Eat nutritious foods, and remember, "garbage in, garbage out."

- Read something every day to inspire, motivate or educate yourself.

- Listen to educational or motivational recordings in your car or through your iPod.

- Select friends and associates with care; conversations and comments heard from the people around you impact your thoughts and the person you become.

- Spend time in silence; turn off the sounds, be still.

- Learn something new; take a course and learn a foreign language or how to play an instrument.

- Conquer one of your fears; improve your public speaking skills, perform in a play or talk to someone new.

Keep exercising your mind. The opportunities are endless and the benefits are amazing. Stimulating your mind with continual learning introduces you to new people, thoughts and ideas. The challenge of doing so improves your life and opens the door to interesting and new opportunities. Are you still growing? Never stop learning or growing as lifelong learning improves more than your mental health.

> *"To do life right, we need to keep learning."*
> — Jane Fonda, American actor

Emotional Fitness

TAKING RESPONSIBILITY FOR YOUR FEELINGS

A friend said to me, "Looking back on my childhood, I don't remember any secrets. I just remember not talking about certain subjects, such as sex, money and religion. My family also had trouble communicating about love, fear, insecurity and anger. Years later, my husband, children and I didn't share at all. We didn't even argue. We thought we were respecting each other by swallowing our thoughts and feelings about potentially hot topics. Actually, we were all emotionally frozen."

> **"The devil made me do it!"**
> — Popularized by Flip Wilson (1933–1998), American comedian and actor

Are you emotionally frozen, or are you aware of your emotions and the variety of emotions you experience? Do you respond to your emotions and feelings in a healthful manner?

Many of us have learned to deny our feelings and rely on our minds' interpretation of the bodily sensations our emotions bring up. We may even rationalize them as being inconsequential or the responsibility of someone else. Instead of being aware of and discussing our feelings, we use words to describe our thoughts. Instead of recognizing the inner source of our feelings by saying, "I feel angry" or "I feel upset," we often say, "I'm so mad at Sam for …" or "You make me upset." We tend to project the source of our emotions onto someone or something else.

When we fail to understand that our feelings come from inside us, we deflect attention away from ourselves and onto another. We deny our responsibility for our feelings and forgo the opportunity to learn about them and the unhealthful ways we often respond to them.

When we respond adversely to our feelings with blame and retribution, we increase the stress levels of all involved, leading to potential alienation. We lose the opportunity to learn, grow and connect better with others and with ourselves. Adverse reactions to emotions are a sign of something being wrong. We need to learn more about their causes.

There is no right or wrong to our feelings, and no one makes us feel a feeling. Our feelings are just that; they are our feelings. They are our personal reactions to a situation. But there is a right way to react to our feelings. Being emotionally frozen is not one of them, nor is reacting adversely as a result of them.

There seems to be a mysterious power attached to our feelings and emotions, a power often marked with a lack of stability, consistency and steadfastness. When we regard our feelings as stronger than we are, similar to saying, "The devil made me do it," we think we get ourselves off the hook for doing something we should not have done. But being ruled by our emotions takes a heavy toll on us and those around us. It weakens us and it also leads to a loss of self-respect.

Webster's describes *emotion* as "a state of feeling" and *feeling* as "an emotional state or reaction." When we react to our feelings, we are responding to something that is forever changing. Some may say we are very emotional, or call us fickle. When we are *fickle*, we are "given to erratic and perverse changeableness" and "marked by lack of steadfastness, consistency or stability."

There are two ways to react to our life experiences. We can react emotionally or intellectually. Emotional reactions include anger, passion and fear. These types of reactions can be erratic. When we react intellectually, we use our knowledge and intelligence to decide how to respond, and we appear rational and confident. When reacting to our feelings, we first make a basic decision. Do we want to be the ruler of our emotions or a slave to them? Do we want to be emotional or intellectual?

We each have a right to our own feelings, but our feelings change. One feeling or another will not last forever. We do not need to react to our feelings in a negative way. We have the ability to choose how we will react. We can say no to them as we learn to understand our emotions and not give in to them. Whether we act on our feelings, cling to them or let them pass, it is within our power and control.

Having accurate definitions for our emotions helps increase our awareness of them and how we respond, thus giving us the power to control them. We can label and deal with what we are aware of. Awareness of and labeling our feelings help us learn to respond in an appropriate manner and build healthier relationships with ourselves and others.

Prior to my diagnosis of major depression and anxiety, I was unaware of the strong feelings I held inside. Through counseling, reading and self-reflection, I came to realize that I carried many unaddressed feelings with me. Feelings of anger, abandonment, rejection, shame and pride were stuffed deep inside. I had not been functioning well or feeling good about myself for some time. I did not like the person I had become.

> *"I am convinced, after many years of ministry that about 85 percent of our problems stem from the way we feel about ourselves."*
>
> — Joyce Meyer, American charismatic, author and speaker

In seeking professional help, I was introduced to a counselor who repeatedly asked me, "How are you feeling today?" But he would not accept "I'm fine," which was the answer I frequently gave him. He continued to push me to be more specific about how I was feeling. I was not familiar with my feelings, nor was I able to label them. You could say I was emotionally frozen. He presented me with a chart similar to the one that follows.

This chart introduced me to a wide variety of feelings. I became aware of what these feelings looked like as I began to label them. I was truly amazed. The only feelings I had previously been aware of were happy, sad and mad. The diagrams on the chart helped me

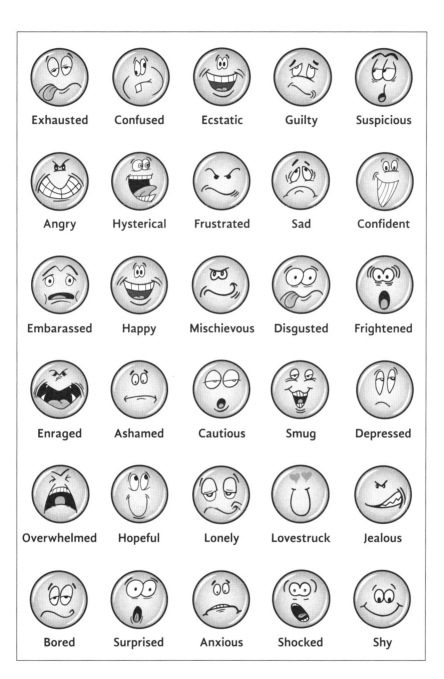

How Are You Feeling Today?

understand and identify how I felt in regards to circumstances in my life, helping me to "defrost" my frozen feelings. I came to understand my feelings and learned that I was not **FINE**, but

- **F**'d up,

- **I**nsecure,

- **N**eurotic, and

- **E**motional.

I was hiding from my true feelings and needed to better understand and express my feelings when asked, "How are you feeling today?" I needed to stop denying my feelings. I began to recognize what I was feeling, learn the causes and then deal with them in an intellectually sound and healthful manner. I did not want to be fickle in responding to my emotions or to what a friend described as all the **ANTS**, or **A**ngry **N**egative **T**hought**S**, crawling around in my head.

I went on to learn that my feelings were a symptom of what was happening in my life and not something to base my responses on. I learned to respond to the intellectual understanding of my feelings, not to the feelings themselves. From there I began to heal from my depression and anxiety. I began to deal with my feelings and my life in a constructive and healthful manner.

Some of us may become emotionally frozen because we have endured pain in the past. We become hard-hearted and bitter. The word *bitter* means something pungent or sharp to the taste. Bitterness can come from small offenses we can't let go of, or the little things we think about over and over again until we've made them monumental in our minds. Bitterness can also result from significant hurts, offenses, traumas or losses we haven't resolved. Bitterness can lead us to turn off our feelings to avoid hurt from reoccurring. It can create walls we believe will protect us, but, actually, they create a self-made prison, keeping people out of our lives as well as pulling us away from experiencing life to its fullest.

Emotional health is a significant and often overlooked aspect of our physical well-being. Our bodies and minds are linked. They are designed to function as an integrated whole to remain healthy.

A meta-analysis of more than 300 scientific articles showed that the expression or repression of emotions has a direct effect on the functioning of our immune systems.[4] The experience of emotions involves a complex release of chemicals affecting all the systems of our bodies.

Disorders found to be related to the repression of our emotional responses include multiple sclerosis, breast cancer and other cancers, inflammatory bowel syndrome, Crohn's disease, ulcerative colitis, gastroesophageal reflux, Alzheimer's disease, asthma, rheumatoid arthritis and rheumatic diseases, as well as depression and anxiety.

In his book *When the Body Says No: Understanding the Disease-Stress Connection*, Dr. Gabor Maté says, "When we have been prevented from learning how to say no, our bodies may end up saying it for us." When we have not learned how to deal appropriately with stressful situations in our lives, our bodies may, in time, find a physical way to deal with them.

In order to heal, we need to feel. Finding effective and appropriate ways to respond to our emotions is critical to maintaining our health. It is part of developing and growing our emotional intelligence.

Dr. Michael Wetter, who served as chief of adult psychiatry at Kaiser Permanente Medical Center in California, explained that by talking through everyday problems and stressors with a friend and sharing our feelings and thoughts, we are able to ward off more serious problems, such as depression and insomnia. When we don't release our feelings regularly, we increase our stress level. Often the physical consequences of our suppressed emotions are worse than the actual stressor.

---

4. Suzanne C. Segerstrom and Gregory E. Miller, "Psychological Stress and the Human Immune System: A Meta-analytic Study of 30 Years of Inquiry," *Psychological Bulletin* 130, no. 4 (2004): 601–630.

When we use our rational and intellectual minds to acknowledge, accept and label the emotions we're feeling, we can use that information to help us decide how to respond. By doing so we learn to understand and calm our emotional responses, slow down and halt the flow of potentially damaging chemicals and give a voice and healthful actions to our emotions.

The length of a roller coaster covers a far greater distance than the distance between where we get on and where we step off. By the time the ride is over, we've spent a great deal of time speeding to great heights and swooping to deep lows. A roller coaster is entertaining, but letting our emotions frequent the roller-coaster ride in everyday life becomes exhausting.

When acting only on emotions, mistakes are often made. Emotions will rise and fall and emotional energy will come and go, rarely leading you in the right direction. Be in charge of your emotions; let them serve you instead of letting them be your master. **A B**etter **C**hoice in responding to your emotions may include the following:

- Let your feelings subside before you decide what to do; wait twenty-four hours—sleep on it.

- Become more aware of your emotions by asking, "**W**hat's **I**mportant **N**ow?" It will help you **WIN** control over your emotions.

- **HALT** when you are **H**ungry, **A**ngry, **L**onely or **T**ired.

- Vent your frustrations to a confidant you feel safe sharing your feelings with, possibly a higher spirit; this takes the pressure off and translates your swirling emotions into coherent thoughts.

- Listen to or read inspirational material to gain insight and wisdom.

- Love yourself and others; this will boost feelings of confidence and security.

- Move around, exercise or get outside.

- Take slow, deep breaths.
- Develop some spiritual practices.

Spiritual Fitness

Spirituality is personal. It is rooted in our connectedness with others and the world around us and is something different for everyone. Spirituality often embraces the concept of searching for the meaning, purpose and direction in life, but doesn't necessarily solve or reach conclusions. It can be a process of self-discovery, whereby we learn who we are and who we want to be. It is questioning and searching for understanding.

"God, grant me the serenity to accept the things I cannot change, the courage to change the things I can, and the wisdom to know the difference."

— Reinhold Niebuhr (1892–1971), American theologian

Spirituality offers many benefits to our lives, emotionally and physically. Connecting with a spiritual side of life gives us time to clear our minds, regain a view of the big picture and look realistically at our achievements and competencies. It gives us time to check the facts, become realistic about a situation and then use our internal values to decide how to respond. Spirituality centers us.

Developing a spiritual practice may help us sort out what we are personally, professionally and socially passionate about, leading to a better understanding of our needs and of what inspires us.

"Nature tops the list of potent tranquilizers and stress reducers. The mere sound of moving water has been shown to lower blood pressure."

— Patch Adams, American physician and speaker

Spirituality is the way some find meaning, hope, comfort and inner peace in their lives. Although spirituality is often associated with religious life, many believe spirituality can be developed outside of a formal religious setting. Acts of compassion and selflessness, altruism and the experience of inner peace are all aspects of spirituality.

Many doctors and scientists are showing an increased interest in the role of spirituality in health and healthcare, perhaps as a result of medical science not having answers to every question about health and well-being. A growing number of studies reveal that spirituality plays a bigger role in the healing process than the medical community had previously thought. Spirituality has even been adopted by the World Health Organization as part of its seven principles of health promotion.

Spiritual practices tend to improve people's coping skills and social support; they promote healthful behavior, reduce feelings of depression and anxiety and encourage a sense of relaxation. By alleviating stressful feelings and promoting healing ones, spirituality can positively influence the immune, cardiovascular, hormonal and nervous systems.

The following questions can assist you in finding a spiritual connection. They are meant to challenge you, reveal gaps in your knowledge and stretch your mind in thinking beyond what has become normal for you. Talk to friends, family or peers about them. Create dialogue to help you figure out what you may not be able to figure out alone. Challenge yourself to be a better person and think about what that means.

- Who are the most important people in my life and how have they affected me?
- With whom do I feel most comfortable?
- If money didn't matter, what would my ideal job be?
- What are my goals for this year? What are my goals for the next five years? Where would I like to be in ten years?
- How do I avoid a stagnant life?
- Do things happen for a reason?

- What are my beliefs about life's purpose?
- What specific experiences have shaped my spiritual beliefs?
- Am I a good person?

Here are some other **TIP**s to evoke a spiritual experience:

- Identify what gives you a sense of inner peace, comfort, strength and connection.
- Be alone; relax and do nothing; reflect and refocus.
- Write in a journal: Be attentive to your emotions as you express feelings and concerns. Write down important moments or thoughts and how certain events, people and things affect your life.
- Meditate: Use music or look at something beautiful, such as sunsets, art or roses. Use relaxation exercises, tapes or visualization techniques.
- Walk or be near the water or nature.
- Do yoga or tai chi as it can create peace within and stimulate your mind.
- Garden: Plant or prune flowers and bushes or pull weeds.
- Clean something.
- Read self-help or spiritual books or biographies.
- Watch movies that move you.
- Do community work: Broaden your understanding of how you fit in with the world, as well as see how others' circumstances differ from your own.
- Pray as a way to find your center, to feel connected and at peace.

Embracing Health, Balance and Abundance with a Fit Body, Mind and Soul

Without a healthy body, mind and soul, you limit who you can be and what you can accomplish.

To fully enjoy life, pursue fitness throughout your entire life. You cannot buy back your health after years of neglect. To be fit, your body requires more than a good exercise and nutrition regimen. You need to be environmentally, mentally, emotionally and spiritually fit because your body houses your physical presence and your spirit. Maintaining a healthy body, mind and soul ensures that your life and your spirit will thrive. To enhance this process in a balanced and healthful way, you may need to **G**et **U**ncomfortable **T**o **S**ucceed. Encourage yourself by saying …

> *"Every human being is the author of his own health and disease."*
>
> — Buddha (c. 563–483 BCE), Indian spiritual teacher

Let It Begin with Me!

Chapter 6

FRIENDS

The Need for Friends

We all need fellowship and community with groups and individuals who offer us encouragement and support. We have a basic need for affection and to engage with like-minded people with similar values. We need someone to believe in us and to associate with people and causes we believe in.

> *"It is a wealthy person, indeed, who calculates riches not in gold but in friends."*
>
> — Jim Stovall, American author and speaker

We enjoy having our work commended, as it confirms belief and faith in ourselves. We benefit from people who commit to an open, honest and accountable relationship with us. To live a healthy, balanced and abundant life, we need people in our lives who think well of us and focus on our better qualities, not on our flaws. We all need friends.

Friendship involves loving and being loved. Friends are people we value. They are our comrades. A friend is someone who is dear to us, someone we want to spend time with and someone we enjoy. Having a friend is to know there is someone at our side, wanting to help and cheer us on as they keep our best interests in mind. Whether they are short-term acquaintances or lifelong companions, friends make life much more abundant.

Friendship has been shown to have a bigger impact on our psychological well-being than family relationships. According to the Mayo Clinic, strong friendships protect us against stress and many forms of mental illness.[1] Dr. Gerald Ellison, director of psychoneuroimmunology at Cancer Treatment Centers of America, Oklahoma, states, "Friends keep us from becoming isolated and lonely; they offer encouragement and support; and they help keep our thinking in line with the real world." He says that when we don't have friends, the isolation and loneliness we experience can lead to illness, discomfort and general ineffectiveness. Friends can also be helpful when we are ill because they offer support and encouragement, which increases hope. Hope has been associated with better immune system function.

> **"Good friends are good for our health."**
>
> — Irwin Sarason (1919–2010), American professor of psychology

Friends plant a hedge of protection around us. Failure to create and maintain quality personal relationships is as dangerous to our physical health as smoking and obesity.

A study of more than 28,000 men found that without strong social ties, they were twenty percent more likely to die ten years sooner, regardless of their health or occupation. The less connected we are, the more prone we are to anxiety, depression, high blood pressure, accidents, suicide and heart disease.[2]

Those lacking strong social support tend to have dramatic and potentially dangerous reactions to worrisome or challenging situations.

---

1. Mayo Clinic staff, "Social Support: Tap This Tool to Combat Stress," *Mayo Foundation for Medical Education and Research* (July 23, 2010), www.mayoclinic. com/health/social-support/SR00033.
2. Patricia M. Enig et al., "Social Ties and Change in Social Ties in Relation to Subsequent Total and Cause-specific Mortality and Coronary Heart Disease Incidence in Men," *American Journal of Epidemiology* 155, no. 8 (2002): 700–709.

The therapy we receive from talking through everyday problems with a friend is priceless. Without this release, the physical toll of our worries and anxieties could be far worse.

While far-off friends may give us health benefits, we need to make sure we have enough face time with closer friends to get the full effect of friendship. Dr. Irene Levine, professor of psychiatry at New York University School of Medicine says, "Cell phones and social media are wonderful for enhancing relationships, but they're not a substitute for face time." It is best to make time to meet our friends in person, even if it means multitasking, getting together to exercise or attending a special event or running errands together. For long-distance friendships, we need to connect in person at least once a year.

As in anything worth having, good friendships take work and time to develop. It takes commitment to build strong, understanding and true friendships.

Choosing your friends wisely helps move your balance wheel of health and well-being through the road of life with greater ease and more fun. Knowing how to identify, create and keep healthy friendships is addressed in the upcoming pages. Being your own best friend, dealing with conflict and finding fulfillment and enjoyment in service work, as well as in your job, are all aspects of friendships. They too are addressed.

BFF: Best Friends Forever

You spend twenty-four hours a day with one person, and that person is you. You wake up every morning with yourself and sleep with yourself every night. It's important to enjoy your own company and be at peace with yourself.

A mark of healthy self-esteem is the ability to spend time alone, without the company of other people. Being comfortable with ourselves and enjoying solitary time reveals inner peace and centeredness. Being alone with ourselves gives us time to listen to our inner callings and needs, which is how we learn and know the person we truly are. Knowing how to nurture ourselves and be our own **BFF**, or **B**est **F**riend **F**orever, is good for our health and well-being.

> *"Don't listen to friends when the friend inside says, 'Do this!'"*
>
> — Mahatma Gandhi (1869–1948), Indian political and spiritual leader

In order to be our own best friend, we need to develop the same kind of tolerant goodwill, positive attitude and love toward ourselves that we feel toward the people we treasure as friends. Knowing how to love and nurture ourselves helps fulfill that need. By giving ourselves the same encouragement, patience and support that a loving parent or friend provides, we learn how to forgive ourselves when we make mistakes and reward ourselves when we do well. This strengthens our physical, mental and emotional health.

To **I**mprove your **P**erformance in being your own **B**est **F**riend **F**orever, consider the following:

- Lift yourself up, don't put yourself down: How you feel about yourself is up to you. If you don't like some of your behavior patterns, change them. If you can't change, accept yourself with love, understanding and compassion. Be aware of your gifts and talents. Let go of your fears and resentments.

- Give yourself positive recognition: When you do something you are proud of, don't let is pass unnoticed; tell yourself you did well.

- Forgive and be compassionate toward yourself: Would your best friend subject you to recrimination for missed opportunities and mistakes made?

- Meet your own expectations: Set reasonable goals for yourself and work toward achieving them while engaging in positive self-talk. Your goals do not need to be grand; minor goals can give you a boost when you allow yourself to savor the success of completion. Be in charge of yourself.

- Get to know yourself better: Fears, desires and fantasies make it hard to see who you really are. The ability to spend time alone in contemplation is important. Self-knowledge helps you become aware and overcome weaknesses that inhibit your happiness, self-respect and success.

- Learn to like and love the person you are.

Ladies, Keep Your Girlfriends

In a lecture called "The Body-Mind Connection: The Relationship Between Stress and Disease," Dr. Alan Schatzberg, a professor of psychiatry at Stanford University, said that one of the best things for a man's health is to be married to a woman, whereas for a woman, one of the best things she can do for her health is to nurture her relationships with her girlfriends.

He went on to say that women connect with each other differently and provide support systems that help each other deal with stress and difficult life experiences. Physically, this quality girlfriend time helps create more serotonin, which is a neurotransmitter needed to combat depression and support a general feeling of well-being.

Women share feelings, whereas men generally form relationships around activities. Men rarely sit down with a buddy and discuss how they feel about themselves or how their personal lives are going. They will talk about jobs, sports, cars, fishing, hunting or golf, but rarely about their feelings.

Women talk about how they feel. They share from their souls. Spending time with a friend is just as important to a woman's general health as jogging or working out at a gym. Women need to talk about what is happening in their lives. So when you hang out with your girlfriend, pat yourself on the back and congratulate yourself for doing something good for your health.

I love my friends and enjoy spending time with them. We take time to listen to each other and give one another support, encouragement and comfort. When I am sad, frustrated, angry or just want to talk, the special connection I've built with my friends is priceless. Speaking with people who understand and want the best for me eases stress, puts a crisis into perspective and allows me to cry and vent openly. My friends also keep me accountable for my actions and responsibilities. I'm very grateful for the outstanding women I call friends.

Pick Your Friends Wisely

> *"Be careful of the environment you choose, for it will shape you; be careful of the friends you choose, for you will become like them."*
>
> — W. Clement Stone (1902–2002), American businessman, philanthropist and author

Think about the friends you have today and people you've known in the past. Some would reliably lift your mood and ease your troubles, but others may have a knack for making you feel worse. Clearly, not all types of friendship are good for your health.

Although we want and need to be accepting of others, we also need a healthy skepticism about human behavior. We are heavily influenced by those around us. When you feel yourself being influenced, proceed with caution. Don't let friends cause you to fail. Many studies show the impact friends have on us. Consider the following findings:

- Friends who talk excessively about others increase our stress.

- Friends can encourage us to make unhealthful lifestyle choices; our risk of becoming overweight increases if a close friend is overweight; the same is true of depression, heavy drinking and smoking.

• Both happiness and unhappiness can spread from one friend to another. Having a happy friend increases the chances of being happy; being surrounded by unhappy friends will drag us down.

A Brigham Young University study used the following quiz in its research to confirm that a strong social network, especially one with healthy friends, improves our chance of living longer by fifty percent.[3]

Consider your group of friends as you take the following quiz and ask, "On the whole, my friends ...

1. Offer constructive help when I have a problem

   Yes ___   No ___

2. Don't insist on getting their own way in everything   Yes ___   No ___

3. Haven't gained a lot of weight recently   Yes ___   No ___

4. Live close enough that we regularly meet face-to-face   Yes ___   No ___

5. Rarely complain of being lonely or tell me they have no one to turn to but me

"Life is too short to spend your precious time trying to convince a person who wants to live in gloom and doom otherwise. Give lifting that person your best shot, but don't hang around long enough for his or her bad attitude to pull you down. Instead, surround yourself with optimistic people."

— Zig Ziglar, American author and motivational speaker

---

3. Julianne Holt-Lunstad, Timothy B. Smith, and J. Bradley Layton, "Social Relationships and Mortality Risk: A Meta-analytic Review," *Public Library of Science Medicine* 7, no. 7 (2010): e1000316, doi: 10:1371/journal.pmed.1000316.

6. Feel happy due to joyful events, such   Yes ____   No ____
   as a son's wedding or finally buying a
   dream home, or just because

7. Always listen with sympathy when I   Yes ____   No ____
   need to vent about work or a vexing
   family situation

8. Feel free to ask me for small favors,   Yes ____   No ____
   such as picking them up at the
   airport or giving them free tax
   advice, and they let me know my
   efforts are appreciated

9. Don't act one way alone with me,   Yes ____   No ____
   but differently in front of others

10. Are not smokers (if even one smokes,   Yes ____   No ____
    count this as a no)

11. May sometimes need my shoulder to   Yes ____   No ____
    cry on, but are ready to return the favor

12. Understand that I'm human and   Yes ____   No ____
    can't always be perfect

13. Lose weight (if needed) by eating   Yes ____   No ____
    right and/or exercising (even if only
    one friend has done this, count this
    as a yes)

14. Try to be tactful and spare my feelings, Yes ____   No ____
    even when they're telling me they
    disapprove of my choices

15. Seem pleased with my relationships   Yes ____   No ____
    and/or family life

16. Almost always answer my calls, show   Yes ___   No ___
    up and make time for me

17. Never stand me up, lie or talk behind   Yes ___   No ___
    my back

18. Have many other friends   Yes ___   No ___

19. Chat back and forth with me (in   Yes ___   No ___
    person, by phone or online) at least
    once a month

20. Make me laugh out loud a lot   Yes ___   No ___

My Score: Total Yes answers _____   Total No answers _____

What Does My Score Mean?

- **More Yes than No answers:** You have health-boosting friends—
  your circle of friends makes you feel connected and needed.

- **About the same number of Yes and No answers:** There is
  room for improvement—your connections could use a checkup,
  as some of your friends may present problems for your
  well-being.

- **More No than Yes answers:** Your circle of friends is in need of
  treatment—you may have landed in this category because,
  although you do have friends, they are not exactly the picture
  of health themselves.

The result of this quiz does not mean you need to drop friends
who stress-eat, drink too much or smoke. The study advises that rather
than focusing on how your friends adversely affect you, concentrate
on how you can affect them for the better. When you improve your
habits, you benefit yourself, and your good example sends healthful
ripples to your friends.

Make sure your chosen relationships push you and your life in the right direction. Put boundaries on relationships. You do not have to do everything your friends do or accept everything they believe in. Keep your eyes fixed on where you want to go and don't be led on a detour that takes you in the wrong direction.

We appreciate one another more if we stay balanced in our relationships. Spending too much time with any one person or a group of people can lead us and them to tire of each other. Don't overdo your relationships with others.

> *"Surround yourself with people most like the person you want to become. Stay away from anyone who can or will bring you down."*
>
> — Tom Hopkins, American author and speaker

The No-Friends-Left (NFL) Club

Would you like to have yourself as a best friend? Are you the type of person you are looking to find as a friend? *To have friends, you need to be a friend.* Do you have the characteristics you want to see in the people you call your friends? Knowing what inhibits the development of friendships is as important as knowing how to develop them.

> *"If you would be loved, love and be lovable."*
>
> — Benjamin Franklin (1706–1790), American scientist and inventor

How we communicate with others will tear down or build our friendships.

- Thoughtless words divide us and they can end relationships and pit us against each other. Idle and hateful words can damage and spread quickly, resulting in pain that is not easy, and often impossible, to undo. Even though we can apologize, scars may remain, destroying a good relationship. Words are like fire; you can neither control nor reverse the damage they do.

- Talking too much and listening too little communicates that our ideas are more important than those of others. Using a mental stopwatch to keep track of how much we talk compared with how much we listen lets others know we value their viewpoints and ideas.

> **"People are lonely because they build walls instead of bridges."**
>
> — Joseph F. Newton, American author

- Judgmental words and thoughts come when we focus on what is wrong with others instead of what is right and good. *Point one finger at another person, then check to see three fingers pointing back at yourself*; this shows that you also have faults.

- Anger damages friendships and our ability to maintain them. When we do not find healthful releases for our anger, we may take it out on those who are close to us. It is OK to be angry, but it is not good to live in anger. It needs to be released in a healthful way. Note that *anger* is one letter short of *danger*. Acknowledging our anger, identifying its source, recognizing our part in it and expressing it lovingly gains respect from others while building friendships.

> **"I don't let my words say nothin' my head can't stand."**
>
> — Louis Armstrong (1901–1971), American jazz trumpeter and singer

- Speak your mind, but criticize the behavior without attacking the person. Remember, *there is no winning an argument, but everyone wins an agreement.* **THINK** and **HALT** and learn to say I'm sorry.

Here are some **TIP**s to improve how you **COMMUNICATE** with friends in ways that build healthier relationships:

- **C**are for and consider others' feelings.
- **O**penness and honesty with others are a must.

- **M**ean what you say and say what you mean.
- **M**utual respect for yourself and others is essential.
- **U**nderstand others' strengths and weaknesses; don't try to change people.
- **N**urture and build your friends' self-esteem and think positively about them.
- **I**ndividuality needs to be cherished so everyone can be themselves.
- **C**larify when you're unsure if what you said or your intention was misunderstood.
- **A**ctively listen to others; especially listen for their feelings.
- **T**rust your friends.
- **E**ncourage and support others in pursuing their goals.

Making New Friends

I've moved to new communities a number of times in my life. These moves created long distances between my friends and me. Even though we remain connected through phone, email and occasional get-togethers, it doesn't feel the same as connecting regularly in person.

To feel connected with others when our friends are not around, going to places where there are crowds, even though they are strangers, can help. Taking public transportation, going to a coffee shop with a good book or your computer, going out to eat or walking along a busy street can help you feel more connected. Creating new friendships and expanding your social network can also be accomplished in the following ways:

- Get out with your pet: Find a popular dog park, stop to chat with the people you meet and make pet playdates.
- Work out: Join a fitness class or start a walking group.

- Just say yes: When you're invited to a party, dinner or other social event, accept the invitation, even if you're tempted to decline.

- Volunteer or join a cause: Strong connections can be formed when you work with people who share a mutual interest or goal. Contact community and volunteer groups such as hospitals, museums, community centers, charitable groups or places of worship.

- Join a hobby group: Consider joining those who have similar interests such as gardening, photography, books or auto racing.

- Go back to school: Add to your knowledge and skills and meet like-minded people at the same time.

- Use social media networks: Social networks can be a fun and free way to play games and meet people with shared interests.

- Hang out on your front porch: Front porches and yards can be neighborhood social centers. Pull up a chair, sit out front with a cup of coffee and a good book; being visible indicates you are friendly and open.

There are many places to meet new people, but creating and maintaining friendships may still be a challenge. Once you have greeted someone new by saying, "Hi," "How's it going?" "What's up?" or "How about this weather?" you can open up the conversation in the following **FORM**:

- **F**amily: "Where are you from?" "Are you married?" "Do you have kids/brothers/sisters?"

- **O**ccupation: "What kind of work do you do?" "Where do you work?" "How long have you been doing that?" "Do you like it?"

- **Re**creation: "Do you have any hobbies?" "Do you play any sports?" "Do you travel?" "Do you enjoy theater, the arts or the museum?"

- **M**essage: A message can be anything you want it to be. Ask what you would like to know: "What room in your house would this painting look the best in?" "Is your company hiring right now?"

Using **FORM** can add excitement to meeting new friends. It indicates that you are interested in the other person and often leads to more interesting conversation. You may find that the most unassuming people have interesting stories and lives, and as you become more familiar with them you can say, "I'd like to talk more. Can we get together for coffee or lunch sometime soon?"

Another **ABC** for creating friendships is to **A**lways **B**e **C**ourteous and to know that the **CORE** ingredients for maintaining friendly relationships are to show **C**ompassion, **O**rderly behavior, **R**espect and **E**mpathy toward others.

To further **I**mprove your **P**erformance in creating and maintaining friendships,

- don't brag, be real and be humble;
- don't tell your problems to everyone;
- don't make excuses;
- admit to your mistakes;
- always talk affirmatively and be positive;
- answer your telephone pleasantly and with a smile on your face; and
- when ridiculed or rejected, treat these as detours, don't take it personally.

Good Conflict

Good communication skills build relationships, whereas negative communication deteriorates relationships and causes conflict. Conflict is inevitable. It happens in our homes, among our friends and colleagues and in our workplaces. It tends to arise because of differing ideas, opinions, needs, beliefs, goals and values.

Conflict costs. It costs us and others on a personal and organizational level. When managed poorly, conflict can take away our happiness, health, productivity and money. Knowing how to manage conflict well or how to engage in effective conflict builds stronger relationships, enhances our productivity and leaves everyone feeling encouraged.

Kenneth Thomas and Ralph Kilmann identified five main styles of dealing with conflict. Each style varies in its degree of cooperativeness and assertiveness, and some styles are more useful than others, depending on the situation. People typically have a preferred conflict-resolution style. Being aware of your preferred style and knowing how to handle conflict effectively and rationally can lead to personal and professional growth, while it builds better friendships and careers. The following table will assist you in knowing your particular conflict resolution style and which style is most effective. (Please see appendix III.)

Conflict-Resolution Styles			
Style	Assertiveness Level	Cooperation Level	When Most Effective
Competing "My way or the highway." FIGHT	High (I win)	Low (You lose)	Quick or unpopular decision required; Protecting self-interest
Avoiding "I'll think about it tomorrow." FLIGHT	Low (Both lose)	Low (Both lose)	Issue is less important; Objective is to diffuse tension

Style	Assertiveness Level	Cooperation Level	When Most Effective
Accommodating "It would be a pleasure." FREEZE	Low (I lose)	High (You win)	Showing reasonableness; Self-sacrifice is OK
Compromising "Let's make a deal." FIFTY-FIFTY	Moderate (Both win and lose)	Moderate (Both win and lose)	Committed to a resolution; Time is constrained
Collaborating "Two heads are better than one." FACE	High (Both win)	High (Both win)	An integrative solution is required; Time is available

Without being consciously aware of conflict-resolution styles, a trigger will set off your habitual reaction. When conflict arises, if your reaction is anger, being judgmental or stewing quietly, chances are you will not feel good about your behavior. **A B**etter **C**hoice is to transform conflict into a positive experience by being aware of and using appropriate negotiation tools:

- Manage your thoughts:
  - Make a conscious choice not to attend the "conflict party."
  - Breathe deeply to relax, giving yourself time to manage your response.
  - Let go of the need to control the other person.
  - Seek first to understand the issue before planning your response.
  - Separate the problem from the person.
  - Name the problem and externalize it.

- Manage your feelings:
  - Continue to breathe deeply to allow your feelings to change.
  - Listen and understand what the other person is saying.

- Manage your body language:
  - Make sure your body language is open, relaxed and nonthreatening.
  - Adjust so you are at eye level with the other person or group.
  - Acknowledge what you are hearing by nodding in an understanding manner.

- Manage your manner of communicating:
  - Speak softly and slowly.
  - Be factual, using "I" rather than "you" statements.
  - Practice active listening.
  - Engage in open dialogue with a goal for understanding the other person.
  - Ask open-ended questions (what? how?).
  - Acknowledge what you are hearing.
  - Affirm you are committed to working through the issue to find the best possible solution.
  - Stay focused on the outcome.
  - Look for underlying issues (differences in goals, opinions, values, needs, ideas).
  - Ask what you can change.
  - Challenge any all-or-nothing thinking.
  - Keep communication on the present with a view to the future.
  - Work together to create a positive outcome.

SERVICE Work: It's in You to Give

Many people build long-term friendships through their involvement in a cause or volunteer work. There is evidence that people who give to others benefit physically and emotionally, and they live longer than those who do not. A Michigan study found that those who did no volunteer work were two-and-a-half times more likely to die during the study than those who volunteered at least once a week.[4]

> *"I don't know what your destiny will be, but one thing I do know: the only ones among you who will be really happy are those who will have sought and found how to serve."*
>
> — Albert Schweitzer (1875–1965), German physician, theologian and philosopher

I've been involved with volunteer organizations and committees for years. Volunteer work helps me learn and know myself better. It takes me out of my comfort zone and introduces me to different people, viewpoints and ways to accomplish things. It gives my life more color and excitement and teaches me to be open to new ideas while overcoming my fears. It brings me new friends and new opportunities.

As we give to others, our giving gives back. Service work helps us to grow and learn more about who we are. It affirms that we have something good to give and gives us the following benefits:

- Physical: Greater longevity, enhanced immune system, decreased stress, lowered cholesterol levels, decreased metabolic rate, improved cardiovascular circulation and healthier sleep

- Emotional: Increased self-acceptance; reduced self-absorption and sense of isolation; expanded sense of control over one's life and circumstances; increased ability to cope with crises;

---

4. Sarah Konrath et al., "Motives for Volunteering Are Associated with Mortality Risk in Older Adults," *Health Psychology* (2011), doi: 10.1037/a0025226.

stronger feelings of personal satisfaction; improved concentration and enjoyment of experiences; enhanced compassion, empathy and sensitivity to others; and reduced inner stress and conflict

- Spiritual: Heightened sense of appreciation and acceptance of others, sustained peace of mind, greater clarity about the meaning and purpose of life, greater connectedness to a higher spirit, more receptivity to spiritual guidance, added involvement in charitable activity and enhanced quality of life

Jalal ad-Din Muhammad Rumi was a thirteenth-century Persian poet and theologian. While addressing our ability to choose what we can do and how to work toward reaching our potential, he told of a man who walked past a beggar. The man asked, "Why, God, do you not do something for these people?" God replied, "I did do something. I made you!"

"There is no exercise better for the heart than reaching down and lifting people up."

— John Andrew Holmes Jr. (1904–1962), American poet and critic

Sherri Ziff Lester, founder of RockYourLife Coaching, says, "There is an indescribable joy we feel when we help someone out or do an unexpected random act of kindness. I call it stepping into the flow of humanity." She says that when we perform random acts of kindness, we receive as we give. When we pass it on, give of ourselves and are thoughtful of others, we feel alive and purposeful.

We feel better about ourselves when we are contributing to the greater good. Through service work we offer **HOPE** by

- **H**elping **O**ther **P**eople **E**xcel,
- **H**elping **O**thers **P**ursue **E**xcellence,

"When people are serving, life is no longer meaningless."

— John W. Gardner (1912–2002), American politician, educator and social activist

- **H**elping **O**ther **P**eople **E**scape, and/or
- **H**elping **O**thers **P**ursue **E**ducation.

Our ability to help others and be involved in some form of service work needs to be promoted. Service work is more than just having something to do. Being involved in service work provides us with a chance to say thank you for the freedom and the abundant lives we are able to live. Whether you volunteer at your local school, coach little league or become part of a neighborhood watch; donate used items or your blood, keep an eye out for a neighborhood senior or become part of your local service club; or help at your church, defend our liberties or teach others how to improve their lives, you are making a difference.

Your help ensures our community and our country are healthy and that they stay healthy and vibrant. Your ideas, leadership abilities, organizational skills and support help find solutions to the issues and concerns facing the people with whom we share our world.

Service work unites us as we work together for a mutual purpose. It brings us new friends, experiences and opportunities for personal growth while we learn to know ourselves better. The circle of giving is never completed without receiving something in return. When you give, you get. Through **SERVICE** you receive

- Self-esteem,

> *"We must delight in each other, make others' conditions our own, rejoice together, mourn together, labour and suffer together, always having before our eyes ... our community as members of the same body."*
>
> — John Winthrop (1588–1649), English lawyer and American colonial governor

> *"Each citizen should play his part in the community according to his individual gifts."*
>
> — Plato (427–347 BCE), Greek philosopher and mathematician

- **E**xperience,
- **R**espect,
- **V**alidation,
- **I**deas,
- **C**onfidence, and
- **E**xcellence.

As with anything you do, receiving the best outcomes requires balance. Volunteering and serving others is no exception. Overcommitting and overextending yourself may lead to stress, setbacks and dissatisfaction. Here is **A B**etter **C**hoice list to manage your volunteerism:

- Do not overextend yourself.
- Do not make promises you cannot keep.
- Do not do it alone.
- Do not overreact.
- Do not be a martyr.
- Do find time to enjoy your work.

"In helping others, we shall help ourselves, for whatever good we give out completes the circle and comes back to us."

— Flora Edwards, American artist

The Joy of Working

We spend more of our waking hours in the office, at the factory, on the road or behind the desk than we do at home. Because of this, it is unfortunate when our attitude toward work is that it is dull, laborious and repetitive, or an irritating necessity of life. With the right attitude, our work, our job, can be so much more.

"The reality is that we are inevitably social creatures who desperately need each other, not merely for sustenance, not merely for company, but for any meaning to our lives whatsoever. These, then, are the paradoxical seeds from which community can grow."

— M. Scott Peck (1936–2005), American psychiatrist and author

In Maslow's hierarchy of human needs, work provides us with the opportunity to meet our physiological needs, and it enables us to meet some of our security and social needs. Yes, work is primarily about obtaining the means to purchase food, shelter and clothing; support our families, friends and others; and entertain and educate ourselves. But our work can also build our self-esteem and be an opportunity to help us reach our potential as we become the people we are meant to be. The list of what our work makes possible is endless.

"What you don't understand is how much pleasure these things can bring you when you have earned them yourself, when leisure becomes a reward for hard work instead of a way to avoid work."

— Jim Stovall, American author and speaker

Work teaches us how to be responsible and adaptable and to take risks. At work we learn how to get along with others, communicate and cooperate. We learn skills and knowledge that we can use at home, in our communities and in other areas of our lives.

At work we can build friendships as we learn to build a positive attitude. What if every day we went to work we grumbled about life from the moment we got there until the moment wc left? Would others want to be around us and talk to us? Would they ask our opinion? Would they ask us to join them for lunch?

"Your work is going to fill a large part of your life, and the only way to be truly satisfied is to do what you believe is great work. And the only way to do great work is to love what you do."

— Steve Jobs (1955–2011), American businessman and inventor

But what if we came to work every day being the positive optimist? Would everybody love us? No, but significantly more people would than if we were the office pessimist. Our attitude toward our work and at our workplaces determines the kind of social environment and the various opportunities we will have the privilege to engage in.

In their book *The Joy of Working*, Denis Waitley and Reni Witt highlight a number of philosophies, or **TIP**s, to create a positive attitude toward work:

> *"Work, supported by a healthy self-image and a positive mental attitude, multiplies all future achievement."*
>
> — Paul J. Meyer, American entrepreneur and author

- Expect the best; eliminate thoughts of the worst that can happen.

- Any problem can be transformed into an opportunity.

- Don't focus on where you came from; focus on where you want to go.

- Learn from your failures as well as your successes.

- Know that success has little to do with outstanding talent, high intelligence or being gifted.

- Life is *ten percent* how you make it and *ninety percent* how you take it.

- Happiness is not something owed to you or handed to you. Happiness is something you make on your own; it's a habit gained from daily practice.

Working with a group of people toward a common goal is exciting. Whether you are bottling pickles on the factory assembly line, laying bricks outside a new home or answering phones at a call center, working together is more fun. As you input numbers on a spread sheet, give needles to relieve pain or direct the activities of a large corporation, when you work together you are part of **TEAM**, where **T**ogether **E**veryone **A**chieves **M**ore. Most often you will find that **T**ogether we create **E**xcellence and **A**lone we create **M**ediocrity.

A healthful work-life balance is also critical to your well-being. Anytime you do too much or too little of something, you become out of balance. Work is no exception. A friend who was a self-proclaimed workaholic explained to me that for years he wasn't balanced in his approach to work; he felt his whole life should revolve around work. He said that as long as he was working and accomplishing something, he didn't feel guilty. But he knew the urge to work all the time was not good for him or his family, and, in time, he began to move toward a more healthful balance in his life. He now says, "Work is a good thing, but I also need to rest and have enjoyment." (Please see appendix III.)

> *"The highest reward for a person's toil is not what they get for it, but what they become by it."*
> — John Ruskin (1819–1900), English critic, essayist and reformer

Embracing Health, Balance and Abundance with Your Friends

Healthy relationships with friends help build self-esteem and confidence. When you have friends around to support and encourage you, life feels good.

You can make new friends by engaging in group activities, service work and employment. In doing so you offer **HOPE** to others while working in a **TEAM**.

It takes time and effort to turn relationships into solid, strong and committed friendships that stand the test of time. Learn to **COMMUNICATE** well as you **FORM** new friendships. Learn how to be a friend, to choose friends carefully and maintain friendships.

It takes being a good friend to have good friends, and you must first remember to be your own **BFF**. But it may take **G**etting **U**ncomfortable **T**o **S**ucceed to create loyal friends. Remember, friendships are set in motion when you say …

Let It Begin with Me!

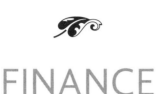

Chapter 7

FINANCE

Financial Health

Money is important. We all need it. Money is the currency we use to buy the basic human needs of food, shelter and clothing. Money also buys the extras. With money we can support our families. We can acquire education, investments and a better life. We can use it to offer help for the greater good. We all need money. But we do not always know how much is enough or how to get it, grow it, keep it safe, have fun with it or give it away.

Just as health and fitness govern our physical lives, money and finances govern our economic lives, but the money we earn and how we manage it also affects our physical health. Money impacts all the other components of our balance wheels of health and well-being. Our **Faith**, **Families**, **Fitness**, **Friends** and **Fun** are all impacted by our **Finances**.

> *"Wealth accumulates when your money is working for you instead of when you're working for your money. It builds systematically over time."*
>
> — Loral Langemeier, American author, speaker and wealth coach

Consider how the following situations would impact your life:

- Being laid off from work and then being unable to find new employment

- Being injured at work and struggling to receive money from Workmen's Compensation or a long-term disability program

- Losing money in the stock market or another investment

- Losing a partner through an accident or illness and not having sufficient insurance or savings to pay your bills or live the life you were accustomed to

- Suffering a relationship breakup, resulting in a decreased standard of living

- Needing to support a child who is in trouble with the law or has extensive disability concerns

- Incurring excessive debt from education, loans, overuse of credit cards or a home purchase

- Entering into a business venture that turned out badly

How would these situations impact the different areas of your life? How would you feel?

Money plays an enormous role in our lives. Financial problems are rated among the highest sources of stress. They lead to unhealthful lifestyles, higher medical needs and an inability to focus. Financial problems cause anxiety, frustration and feelings of hopelessness, often accompanied by substance abuse, overeating, cardiovascular disease, stomach disorders and more. The resulting stress, anxiety and lack of sleep can bring about minor illnesses and exacerbate existing conditions, including depression, back pain, headaches, asthma and cancer. Financial troubles can be overwhelming and all consuming, leading to moodiness and generally feeling run down.

A 2005 study exploring the negative health effects of financial stress lists numerous physical and mental health conditions that result from financial distress.[1] A 2011 study concluded that financial strain places some individuals at increased risk of engaging in addictive behaviors.[2]

When we have financial problems, we are more likely to neglect our health. We may buy unhealthful food and be physically inactive, resulting in health problems that lead to absenteeism at work, which, in turn, leads to greater financial problems. Stress from financial worries creates a poor attitude at work as we may be less focused, unproductive or careless, risking our job security.

When we are in control of our finances and free of financial burdens, we have peace of mind. Our overall health, attitude, performance and ability to focus improve.

Many of us have surprisingly little knowledge about how to manage money, and it may be a difficult subject to talk about. We often do not know what questions to ask or whom to ask. We may not want someone else to know our financial situation or how poor our knowledge of financial management truly is. We avoid conversations about money because it may elicit emotions of fear, anger, envy or greed. Money is one of the main causes of divorce, but couples avoid talking about money for fear of creating conflict.

How often do we share our financial health and challenges with our healthcare professional? If we did, perhaps the best prescription would be to seek the aid of a financial advisor—an accountant, financial planner, insurance advisor, lawyer or tax advisor well versed in their trade and sensitive to supporting our financial dilemmas.

As a nurse, I am not qualified to give financial advice. So in this chapter I will share some basics about financial health and encourage

---

1. Barbara O'Neill, Benoit Sorhaindo, Jing Jian Xiao, and E. Thomas Garman, "Negative Health Effects of Financial Stress," *Consumer Interests Annual* 51 (2005), www.personalfinancefoundation.org/research/efd/Negative-Health-Effects-of-Financial-Stress.pdf.
2. Benjamin A. Shaw, Neda Agahi, and Neal Krause, "Are Changes in Financial Strain Associated with Changes in Alcohol Use and Smoking among Older Adults?" *Journal of Studies on Alcohol and Drugs* 72, no. 6 (2011): 917–925.

you to seek out the help and information you need to build and strengthen your financial health and well-being. Being financially fit, like being physically fit, happens when you have the desire to improve yourself and use the proper techniques and strategies to do so.

What's Your KASH Flow?

Learning to manage our money ensures we have sufficient financial resources to meet our daily and future needs. It provides us with the opportunity to purchase healthful food and engage in sports and other physical activities. It gives us time to spend with our families and friends, take vacations and educate our children. It helps us acquire sufficient funds for a comfortable retirement. A healthy cash flow enables us to afford the essentials of life with some extra to have healthy, balanced and abundant lifestyles.

In his book *Safari to the Soul*, Denis Waitley discusses the **KASH**-flow of life, an acronym that helps you understand and implement effective money-management strategies. When your financial **K**nowledge, **A**ttitudes, **S**kills and **H**abits are strong, so are your well-being and the lives of those you love.

- **K**nowledge: Money is a tool, and learning to handle it unemotionally and effectively is wise. Improving your knowledge of how money works puts you in control of your finances.

- **A**ttitudes: A positive attitude toward money puts you in the black, whereas a negative attitude may put you in the red. What is your attitude toward money? Do you see money as the root of all evil or as a vehicle for a better life? Being critical or envious of those with more money than you wastes energy and decreases your ability to focus on your own needs. Fearing money and your responsibility toward it makes it difficult to manage it effectively.

- **S**kills: You improve your financial skills by observing, imitating and doing. Building better skills in managing a budget, controlling your spending and investing results in increased income, confidence and success.

- **H**abits: You may need to discard some of your spending and money-management habits and replace them with those that increase your cash flow. The more you train, the more you gain. A step-by-step approach can help you reach your goals. Practice makes perfect, and it makes permanent.

Developing the required **K**nowledge, **A**ttitudes, **S**kills and **H**abits to build your financial acumen and bank account takes time. It may require you to go back to school or receive some formal training to advance your skill set. You may need to work for awhile at a job you do not like or for a boss whom you are not fond of. You may need to spend a few years during which you do not have much excess cash. Preparation and time are key components to improving your **KASH** flow.

Some basic **TIP**s **T**o **I**mprove your **P**erformance in obtaining Financial Health include these fundamental principles of money management:

- There is no free lunch.
- Money doesn't grow on trees.
- A penny saved is a penny earned.
- Wealth doesn't accumulate until debt is eliminated.
- Live below your means.
- Wants are not needs.
- If it's too good to be true, it probably isn't true.
- It takes money to make money.
- Money is not evil, but hoarding it is.

- Share your wealth, as giving will pay back huge dividends.
- Credit card interest charges are a bad sign.
- Payday loans are worse than credit cards.

Engaging the expertise, support and guidance of financial advisors who are good teachers and see your financial health from a holistic perspective will ensure you reach your **KASH** flow goals sooner and with greater peace of mind.

Do You Have PMS?

What is your relationship with money? What does money mean to you? What drives you when it comes to money?

Some people are critical of those who earn high incomes, claiming unfairness, yet they do not work hard or develop the skills and habits required to gain financial independence and security for themselves. Some may even believe that those who are financially secure and independent are just **LUCK**y. But it is by **L**aboring **U**nder the **C**orrect **K**nowledge of managing and growing money that most successful people reach financial security and independence. Becoming financially fit requires a positive mind-set, and eliminating any "scarcity mentality," or **P**overty **M**entality **S**yndrome (**PMS**), we may have.

Some of us grew up in households where finances were discussed. Others grew up in homes where money was never spoken about openly. In some families and social circles, discussing personal finances may be considered to be rude and a taboo subject, whereas in others it is perfectly acceptable. Our early conditioning and environments play a role in determining our attitude toward money, as many of our financial habits and attitudes are influenced by our parents.

If your parents believed they had to work hard for their money, you may believe the same. If your parents believed it is unwise to spend money on anything "extra," this too would affect your attitude. Other attitudes that demonstrate a scarcity mentality include the following:

- I don't believe in money.
- Money is dirty.
- You must sell your soul for money.
- Money is the root of all evil.
- Never dip into your savings.
- We can't afford it.
- I don't want to spend the money.
- I don't deserve it.

A family member needed to buy a new pair of shoes to replace the worn-out pair he wore daily in his work in sales, but he said, "I can't buy new shoes. I'm broke!" He made enough money to meet more than his basic needs, and yet I often heard him say this, so I asked, "Why do you always say you're broke?"

He said, "I'm cheap! I have the money, but I just don't want to spend it!" So I said, "You have **PMS**."

> *"Poverty is untested potential."*
> — Denis Waitley, American motivational speaker and author

Thinking and speaking negatively about money and our finances diminishes our financial well-being. However, when we say, "I can buy what I need in life," "I am careful with my spending habits" and "I am thankful for the money I have," we demonstrate a positive attitude toward our finances. This attitude, along with the right knowledge, skills and habits, goes a long way to building financial well-being.

Remember, you become the person you think you are. People who think of themselves as poor will be poor, just as people who consider themselves failures will fail. Those who think of themselves as successful and wealthy find the opportunities to achieve success and wealth!

How Much Money Passes through Your Hands?

"Don't tell me where your priorities are. Show me where you spend your money and I'll tell you what they are."

— James W. Frick, American politician

Have you ever thought about the amount of money that will pass through your hands during your lifetime? How much money will you earn during your working career?

The following table shows how different levels of monthly income accumulate over ten, twenty, thirty and forty years. (Note: The figures represent income only; investment income is not taken into account.)

Accumulation of Monthly Income over the Years				
Monthly Income	10 Years	20 Years	30 Years	40 Years
$2,000	$240,000	$480,000	$720,000	$960,000
$4,000	$480,000	$960,000	$1,440,000	$1,920,000
$6,000	$720,000	$1,440,000	$2,160,000	$2,880,000
$8,000	$960,000	$1,920,000	$2,880,000	$3,840,000
$10,000	$1,200,000	$2,400,000	$3,600,000	$4,800,000
$15,000	$1,800,000	$3,600,000	$5,400,000	$7,200,000

How much of your monthly income will you save and grow through the years? Thomas Stanley and William Danko, marketing professors and researchers, surveyed millionaires. In their books *The Millionaire Next Door* and *Stop Acting Rich … and Start Living Like a Real Millionaire*, they found that many wealthy people live in middle-income neighborhoods, drive economical cars, wear simple watches and buy their suits off the rack.

They also found other **TIP**s that enhance the financial security of the wealthy:

- Income does not equal wealth: The size of one's paycheck is only thirty percent of what creates wealth; what matters is how much income is invested. On average, millionaires invest nearly twenty percent of their income.

- Work that budget: The majority of millionaires create a budget they follow.

- Know where your dough goes: Almost sixty-five percent of the wealthy answer yes to the question, "Do you know how much your family spends each year for food, clothing and shelter?" Wealthy people are more likely to keep track of their spending.

- Know where you want your dough to go: Two-thirds of millionaires answered yes to, "Do you have a clearly defined set of daily, weekly, monthly, annual and lifetime goals?"

- Time is money: The wealthy take time to goal plan, spending nearly twice as many hours per month planning their investments compared with those with less wealth. Most wealth accumulators use a regimented schedule to plan their investments.

- Love the home you are in: Half of millionaires live in the same house for more than twenty years. Choice of home and neighborhood greatly impacts wealth and consumption; for example, living in a high-priced home in an exclusive community increases spending and impairs the ability to save.

- Love the spouse you are with: The majority of wealthy people are married and stay married to the same person. A study by an Ohio State University researcher showed that a person who marries and stays married accumulates nearly twice as much personal wealth as a person who is single or divorced. Those who divorce lose, on average, three-quarters of their personal net worth. Marrying someone with disciplined financial habits is also important. In the majority of millionaire households studied, the husband was the main breadwinner and tended to be frugal, but the wife was even more frugal.[3]

- Don't drive away your wealth: The majority of millionaires own their cars rather than lease them and drive cars four years old or older. One-third buy used vehicles.

- The rich are different; they are happier: Living below your means and having money in the bank brings peace of mind. Financially independent people do not seek status purchases to improve their happiness.

> *"It's good to have money and the things that money can buy, but it's good, too, to check up once in a while and make sure that we haven't lost the things that money can't buy."*
>
> — George Horace Lorimer (1867–1937), American journalist, author and editor

How Much Money Is Enough?

Knowing what is important in our lives and keeping our priorities in perspective helps us know how much money is enough. A large bank account in itself does not equate to abundance. Our society tends to revere money and material things, but they need not be made our top priority.

Understanding what you want from life is the first step to laying the foundation for financial planning. Knowing what you value, where you want to go and what you want to accomplish must guide your choices, especially your educational and financial choices.

The following story illustrates how two people who ultimately share the same values and goals for their life make different choices on how to obtain them.

---

3. Jay L. Zagrosky, "Marriage and Divorce's Impact on Wealth," *Journal of Sociology* 41, no. 4 (2005): 406–424.

The Fisherman

A businessman was at the pier of a coastal Mexican village, when a fisherman in a small boat docked. Inside the small boat were several large tuna. The businessman complimented the Mexican on the quality of his fish and asked how long it took to catch them. The Mexican replied, "Only a little while."

The businessman asked, "Why don't you stay out longer and catch more fish?"

"I have enough to support my family's immediate needs," replied the fisherman.

"What do you do with the rest of your time?" asked the businessman.

The fisherman replied, "I sleep late; fish a little; play with my children; take a siesta with my wife, Maria; and stroll into the village each evening, where I sip wine and play guitar with my amigos. I have a full and busy life, Señor."

The businessman scoffed, "I am a Harvard MBA and I could help you. You need to spend more time fishing, and with the proceeds, buy a bigger boat. With the proceeds from the bigger boat you could buy several boats; eventually you would have a fleet of fishing boats. Instead of selling your catch to a middleman, you would sell directly to the processor and eventually open your own cannery. You would control the product, processing and distribution. You would need to leave this small coastal fishing village and move to Mexico City, then LA, and eventually New York City, where you would run your expanding enterprise."

"But Señor, how long will this all take?" asked the fisherman.

"Fifteen to twenty years," said the businessman.

"But what then, Señor?"

The businessman laughed and said, "That's the best part! When the time is right, you sell your company to the public and become very rich. You would make millions."

"Millions, Señor? Then what?"

"Then you would retire, move to a small coastal fishing village where you would sleep late, fish a little, play with your kids, take a siesta with your wife, stroll to the village in the evenings where you could sip wine and play your guitar with your amigos."

The fisherman, smiling, said, "Isn't that what I'm doing right now?"

— **Author unknown**

It is difficult to put together a sound financial plan for your life without first knowing what you really want, and what is really important to you. If security, more time with family and friends, being less rushed and less busy, living longer and making a difference by helping others are important to you, but you are living paycheck to paycheck, something is wrong with your financial plan.

"Financial Security is that amount of assets that will give you a specific income, after taxes, to live like you want to, without having to depend on day-to-day employment."

— Denis Waitley, American motivational speaker and author

Money is simply a tool, and as with any tool, you need to learn how to use it correctly and for the right purpose. Money is a piece of paper that represents value. It can be used for good or for evil, or it can be left idle. Essential to using money correctly and for the right purpose is to understand what money means to you and to know how much money is enough for you.

Real financial security is a state of mind, which is only partially dependent on the size of our bank account. Financial security comes from our understanding of security and how we deal with the ideas that cause us to feel insecure.

If you have $2,000,000 in the bank and you make a substantial six-figure income, yet feel you need to keep up with your super-wealthy friends, you may find yourself spending $300,000 a year or more and feeling miserable and financially insecure.

On the other hand, if your income is $5,000 a month and you spend $4,600 and save $400 each month, and you are involved with your family and friends and busy with activities and hobbies, you can feel happy and financially secure. You have enough.

People with less money have different lifestyles than those with more money, but does a cold beer really taste better at a fancy resort than it does in your backyard with close friends? Does billionaire Bill Gates get more pleasure from his morning coffee and crossword puzzle than you do from yours?

Money can buy medicine but not health.
Money can buy a house but not a home.
Money can buy companionship but not friends.
Money can buy entertainment but not happiness.
Money can buy food but not an appetite.
Money can buy a bed but not sleep.

— Author unknown

LUCK Improves Your Financial Well-Being

In his book *How Rich People Think*, Steve Siebold says, "When it comes to spending money to enrich our life, education should be a greater priority than entertainment." He says the more financially successful people become, the more successful they believe they can become. He suggests we put our money toward classes, seminars and books that teach us how to be successful.

Reading will give you knowledge,
Action will give you experience,
Results will give you confidence.

— Loral Langemeier, American author,
speaker and wealth coach

In 1930, George Samuel Clason published *The Richest Man in Babylon*. Since then, his book has become a classic and has been acclaimed as "the greatest of all inspirational works on the subject of thrift and financial planning." Clason's book offers financial advice through allegorical stories or parables set in ancient Babylon. The characters, and thus the readers, learn universal principles about how to avoid debt, seek financial mentors and protect their assets.

The book explains how to build a good foundation for financial success. Its timeless wisdom is simple, direct and effective. In the parable "Seven Cures for a Lean Purse," Clason offers financial principles for increasing our **LUCK** with money. It offers us guidance so we can **L**abor **U**nder **C**orrect **K**nowledge. The seven cures give insight into wealth-building and the concept that money is plentiful for those who understand the simple rules of its acquisition. Following are the concepts Clason promotes through the seven cures:

"The first cure I did discover for my lean purse: 'For each ten coins I put in, to spend but nine.'"

— George Samuel Clason (1874–1957), American soldier, businessman and author

1. START THY PURSE TO FATTENING

No matter how much money flows through your hands, you cannot achieve financial independence without knowing how to pay yourself first. If you put ten apples in a basket every morning and every evening you remove nine, the basket will soon be overflowing with apples. The same happens when you save ten percent of your income. No matter how much it is, over time, your bank account will grow to overflowing.

Setting aside ten percent of your income before all other expenses are considered accomplishes that overflow. Before you commit your money to living expenses, and before you buy any "toys," take out ten percent and live on nine-tenths of your income. Always live on less money than you make. You may say, "But how can I live on nine-tenths, when I can't live on ten-tenths?" The reply is, "It's not going to make much difference."

You will never accumulate wealth and gain financial independence if you live your life paycheck to paycheck. When you live that type of lifestyle, your **JOB** is keeping you **J**ust **O**ver **B**roke. If you always pay yourself first, you create a lifelong savings plan. You can build your estate, retirement fund and your children's education fund and acquire the ability to sustain yourself and your family for months, and even a lifetime, without worry.

2. CONTROL THY EXPENDITURES

A key to implementing effective money-management habits is to differentiate between necessities and desires. Buying everything we want leaves no money to save, grow and invest. Maintaining a weekly, monthly and yearly budget for money we

> *"Budget thy expenses that thou mayest have coins to pay for thy necessities, to pay for thy enjoyments and to gratify thy worthwhile desires without spending more than nine-tenths of thy earnings."*
>
> — George Samuel Clason

need to allocate to household expenses keeps us organized and on track.

There are many budgeting forms and templates available on the Internet, in books, at banks or from financial advisors. Take the time to complete an income and expense sheet and then maintain it monthly. This is the beginning of a solid financial plan.

> *"It is human nature to want it and want it now; it is also a sign of immaturity."*
>
> — Dave Ramsey, American financial author and speaker and radio and television personality

Warren Buffett, one of the richest men in the world, still lives in the house he bought in 1958 for $31,500, and Ingvar Kamprad, owner of IKEA, still drives a fifteen-year-old car and flies economy class.

The amount of money you make is important, but it is secondary to the degree to which you control what you spend. Budgeting and planning your expenses diligently is what truly counts in money management. Ask yourself if the purchase is absolutely necessary.

It may be difficult to identify necessary expenses, because they seem to grow in proportion to our incomes. When we earn more, we seem to need more—unless we put up a stop sign to our desires. Spending on a little luxury isn't bad, as long as we budget for these extras without spending more than ninety percent of our income.

Remember to let your emotions subside before you decide to make a purchase. It is amazing what a difference twenty-four to forty-eight hours can make. Learn to wait, even when it's on sale.

3. MAKE THY GOLD MULTIPLY

Setting aside ten percent of your income and living off ninety percent is the foundation for becoming financially secure and independent, but it is not enough. The money you save needs to be put to work in order to produce more money.

Everything you save should earn some-thing. Money grows when you invest it; it multiplies by compounding your returns. When you put your savings to work, it collects interest and builds income streams. The interest is then added to the principal to earn more interest.

Which would you choose—to be given a million dollars today or a penny that doubles itself each day for a month? If you choose the penny that doubles itself daily, you will have considerably more money in thirty days. You will have $5,368,710. That's the wonder of compound interest.

> *"To put each coin to laboring that it may reproduce its kind, even as the flocks of the field, and help bring to thee income, a stream of wealth that shall flow constantly into thy purse."*
>
> — George Samuel Clason

That's where **LUCK** comes in. Understanding compound returns and incorporating it into your financial strategy increases your wealth.

With education and understanding, you can safely invest your money by striving for a reasonable risk-reward ratio. You may find it difficult to take calculated investment risks for fear of losing money. This is understandable. But remember, money in your pocket earns you nothing.

In addition, many people who dream of financial security fantasize about inheriting money or winning a lottery. Dreaming does little to build financial security. Some will spend $10 to $30 a week on lottery tickets, adding up to $520 to $1,560 a year that could be used to invest. The dollars spent on lottery tickets could provide a steady return of income for future use when those same dollars are put to work in sound financial investments.

4. GUARD THY TREASURES FROM LOSS

When buying a second-hand car, what do you do? You check out the car, test drive it, inspect it, apply for the Vehicle History Report and

> *"Guard thy treasure from loss by investing only where thy principal is safe, where it may be reclaimed if desirable, and where thou will not fail to collect a fair rental. Consult with wise men. Secure the advice of those experienced in the profitable handling of gold. Let their wisdom protect thy treasure from unsafe investments."*
>
> — George Samuel Clason

> *"Every man can be wealthy; he just needs the right navigator."*
>
> — Melvin Kaspardlov (1924–1995), Canadian radiologist

ask a friend who is more of an expert than you before deciding to part with your money. The same applies to investments. Don't put money into an investment without doing proper research.

Warren Buffett has two rules for investing. The first is to never lose money, and the second is to always remember rule number one. When you are ready to invest, make sure you have educated yourself. Learn from experienced financial advisors and those who know their trade well, but remember, only you can keep your best interests at the forefront; take control of that responsibility.

Further **TIP**s for guarding your treasure: Be wary of

- "hot tips" and promises of astronomical returns,
- start-up businesses in the classified ads,
- unrealistic expectations,
- investments you are not familiar with, and
- lending money to family and friends.

5. MAKE OF THY DWELLING A PROFITABLE INVESTMENT

Home ownership is preferable to renting. At some point, mortgage payments end and home ownership is achieved. Although owning a home has many benefits, there are certain factors you need to be aware of. Owning a home includes financial responsibilities that, if not handled properly, can make your home a liability, not an asset. Don't become house poor. Consider the cost of maintenance, utilities, taxes and other fees.

Learn strategies to pay off your mortgage quickly. Some mortgage strategies to become debt-free faster include the following:

- Make sure your down payment is large enough to minimize mortgage interest rates and fees.

- Consider paying mortgage payments weekly or bi-weekly instead of monthly.

- Endeavor to pay an extra five to ten percent in principal each year.

- Wait to renovate.

> *"Thus come many blessings to the man who owneth his own house. And greatly will it reduce his cost of living, making available more of his earnings for pleasures and the gratification of his desires. This, then, is the fifth cure for a lean purse: Own thy own home."*
>
> — George Samuel Clason

6. INSURE A FUTURE INCOME

The future is unknown, but you can take steps to protect yourself, your family and your financial security from disability, illness and death. In *Smart Couples Finish Rich*, David Bach lists the following ways to protect your financial well-being and future income from unforeseen circumstances:

> *"Provide in advance for the needs of thy growing age and the protection of thy family."*
>
> — George Samuel Clason

- Save at least three and up to twenty-four months' worth of living expenses in case of emergency.

- Have an up-to-date will.

- Have adequate life insurance coverage and consider the importance of critical-illness and disability insurance.

- Consider long-term-care coverage, especially when you are over sixty.

"Thus the seventh and last remedy for a lean purse is to cultivate thy own powers, to study and become wiser, to become more skillful, to so act as to respect thyself. Thereby shalt thou acquire confidence in thy self to achieve thy carefully considered desires."

— George Samuel Clason

7. INCREASE THY ABILITY TO EARN

Charles Schwab, an icon in the financial world and author of *Charles Schwab's Guide to Financial Independence*, says he has a "terrible bias" about where people should make their initial financial investment. "I really think people should make their first investment in themselves." Invest in yourself and in your life through education.

Education does not need to be formal. There are many successful people who have accumulated their wealth without obtaining formal education. In fact, the cumulative wealth of successful people who do not have a college or university education actually greatly outnumbers those who do.

Bill Gates, Steve Jobs and Mark Zuckerberg all dropped out of school, but they never stopped learning and improving their knowledge. Learning happens by observing others, through our life experiences and through a commitment to continue to learn. We can learn and continue to learn by reading, attending workshops and seminars and seeking the advice of those who are more skilled than we are. When we have the desire, we can learn what we need to become wealthy and successful.

If you are not earning the money you want or think you deserve, consider the following choices:

- Develop new skills in your area of employment.

- Take on more important tasks at work.
- Take a second or part-time job.
- Turn a favorite hobby or skill into extra income.
- Increase your capabilities and knowledge through further education.

Staying Debt-Free

Clason's seven cures provide the tools needed to build wealth. But building wealth and financial security cannot happen as long as debt exceeds our wealth-generating assets. Eliminating debt does not happen immediately, and to do so may require breaking money habits that reflect past conditioning and old thinking. In the end, the only way to get out of debt is to stop spending money and rebuild. There are many resources to help, such as asking your financial advisor or searching out a debt-management company.

> *"If someone is going down the wrong road, he doesn't need motivation to speed him up. What he needs is education to turn him around."*
>
> — Jim Rohn, (1930–2009), American entrepreneur, author and motivational speaker

In *The Total Money Makeover*, David Ramsay says, "Debt has been sold to us so aggressively, so loudly, and so often that to imagine living without debt requires myth-busting." He goes on to say that debt has become so ingrained in our culture that most people cannot imagine, let alone consider, having a car without a payment, a house without a mortgage, being a student without a loan or having credit without a credit card balance. Most people cannot envision what life would be like with no loan payments.

> *"The rich rule over the poor and the borrower is the slave of the lender."*
>
> — Proverbs 22:7

Debt is insidious. It is subtle, but it can mean the difference between living forever in a rented apartment or building wealth by purchasing a home with a good mortgage interest rate. It can mean the difference between driving a reliable new-model car and taking the bus to work. It can mean the difference between staying at home for vacations and traveling to see the wonders of the world.

Debt can cause you to become discouraged and depressed, but learning ways to eliminate and avoid debt enhances your life and reduces your stress. Making conscious decisions about how you want to manage your money, staying committed to reaching your financial goals and doing what you need to do to reach them means you may need to **G**et **U**ncomfortable **T**o **S**ucceed. Purchases held off because they are only wants give you peace of mind and a sense of security. Disciplined spending is investing today to reap benefits tomorrow.

As you work to eliminate your debt, be aware there is good debt and bad debt. In *The Fireman and the Waitress*, Dessa Kaspardlov, a financial planner, highlights three points to avoid getting caught in the debt trap:

1. Incurring debt just because you want to purchase a new set of high-end golf clubs as a birthday gift for yourself is bad debt.

2. Incurring debt to acquire wealth, such as a mortgage on your own home is good debt.

3. Leveraging or incurring debt to earn income and get a tax refund or borrowing to invest wisely is good debt.

Teach Your Children to Be Self-Supporting

When financial issues are kept hidden and discussions about money are not encouraged, children in the household suffer. If finances are not openly discussed, poor habits may be learned from family and friends and those not qualified to teach healthy finances.

Teaching children financial responsibility—how to appreciate and handle money—is an important responsibility for parents. The lessons we teach our children about money management will help them throughout life. We will not need to worry about them, and they will not become a financial burden.

When we teach our children about finances, we need to explain the consequences of not working and let them know what it feels like to not have enough money. Teach them how to buy what they need rather than what they want. This lays the foundation for understanding that money does not come in limitless amounts without putting in the effort to obtain it; they cannot simply manufacture money or use credit when they don't have it. Teaching our children how to earn money by giving them opportunities to work for it will go a long way toward helping them become self-supporting.

Providing children with an allowance is a common practice in many families, but they really don't need one. Chores are considered one of the responsibilities of being part of a family. Instead of an allowance, offer your children extra jobs that they are paid to do so they understand the work it takes to earn money. In this way, they learn to appreciate the value of the money they have and are better able to manage it wisely.

> "The worst thing you can do is never talk about money with your family. The best thing a parent—or marriage partner, for that matter—can do is say it is OK to talk about money: how to handle it, manage it, save it, budget it."
> — Charles R. "Chuck" Schwab, American stock brokerage pioneer

> "As adults, our conditioning is so ingrained ... If we want to adopt something new, we've got to change our mind. Kids are in a great position because they're just making up their mind."
> — Bob Proctor, Canadian author, speaker and coach

A colleague once explained to me that his children did not receive an allowance because he and his wife believed an allowance was similar to a handout or subsidy. They wanted their children to understand that they must work to earn money, so they provided opportunities for them to earn money through work assignments.

Each child had a weekly assignment sheet with five household chores they were expected to do, such as cleaning their bedroom or putting away the dishes. The parents paid $1 for each chore. There were also bonus assignments, so the children had the opportunity to earn extra money.

As it turned out, one of his children was very good at completing his assignments, whereas another occasionally slipped up. When she saw her brother earning more, she learned a valuable lesson about completing her work. The experience did not upset the children or hinder their growth; in fact, they learned many valuable lessons.

When my colleague first started the work-assignment routine with his children, he said they regularly spent their earnings on inexpensive toys, but soon learned that if they saved their money, they could purchase higher-quality items they valued more.

These parents also gave each child three envelopes labeled "Giving," "Saving" and "Spending." As soon as the children were paid, they would place a dollar of their income in the Giving envelope and then divide the rest between their Saving and Spending envelopes. This taught them the importance of balance in their lives and not spending everything they earned. Teaching children to give some of their money away keeps them from becoming greedy and builds generosity in their hearts.

It is never too late to teach children about financial responsibility, although the earlier the better. Teaching our children basic money-management skills allows them to be financially self-supporting and secure—not financially strapped later on and needing their parents' support in adulthood.

Embracing Health, Balance and Abundance with Financial Fitness

No matter what you do to build financial security, you will improve your **LUCK** when you learn to **L**abor **U**nder **C**orrect **K**nowledge. You will enhance your **KASH** flow when you build your **K**nowledge, **A**bilities, **S**kills and **H**abits. All this will take time, energy and the right attitude.

Learning to budget your money, save it, invest it wisely and say no to unnecessary wants takes **G**etting **U**ncomfortable **T**o **S**ucceed. It takes **GUTS** to discipline yourself to incorporate wealth-building strategies into your life. It is also a skill and a habit that requires you to constantly say to yourself ...

Let It Begin with Me!

Chapter 8

DEATH AND TAXES

While planning this book, I struggled with where I would introduce the topic of death and dying. After reading Benjamin Franklin's quote, I knew. As paying taxes are a part of financial fitness, and taxes and death are certainties of life, it seemed fitting to address death and dying after discussing finance.

> **"In this world nothing can be said to be certain, except death and taxes."**
>
> — Benjamin Franklin (1706–1790), American scientist and inventor

I also struggled with which aspects of death and dying to bring forward in this chapter. I decided to begin with how we talk about death and dying, then address the dying experience and move on to hospice palliative care and the sustaining of life. I introduce leaving a legacy of our lives, which leads to giving at death, and to taxes. At the end I discuss the taxes we pay while we're living.

Talking about Death and Dying

Many will remember the 1998 comedy *Patch Adams* starring Robin Williams. It is based on the life of Hunter Doherty "Patch" Adams, an American physician, social activist and author. In his book *Gesundheit: Good Health Is a Laughing Matter*, Patch describes death as

To die. To expire. To pass on. To perish. To peg out. To push up daisies. To push up posies. To become extinct. Curtains, deceased, demised, departed and defunct. Dead as a doornail. Dead as a herring. Dead as a mutton. Dead as nits. The last breath. Paying a debt to nature. The big sleep. God's way of saying slow down.

> *"The trouble with quotes about death is that 99.999 percent of them are made by people who are still alive."*
>
> — Joshua Bruns

> *"For everything there is a season, a time for every activity under heaven. A time to be born and a time to die. A time to plant and a time to harvest."*
>
> — Ecclesiastes 3:1–2

Patch defines death with lightness and humor. He brings it into the open, reinforcing that it is a normal part of life. Life is unpredictable. We do not know what turns it will take or how fast it will go. We only know death is certain. It is a part of life, a part of nature and of our biology. Everything that lives eventually dies. Plants and animals die. People die.

A study from the University of Bradford in the United Kingdom explored views of dying, death and bereavement from family members of people who died from heart failure. The researchers discovered most people find end-of-life discussions with their loved ones to be difficult.[1] It appears we can make light of death when it is further away from us, but as it comes closer, we shy away from it.

Are you afraid of dying? Are you afraid of the loss that will occur when a loved one

---

1. Neil Small et al., "Dying, Death and Bereavement: A Qualitative Study of the Views of Carers of People with Heart Failure in the UK," *BMC Palliative Care* 8, no. 6 (2009), doi:10.1186/1472-684X-8-6.

dies? Do you think not talking about death keeps it at a distance?

Whatever we think and feel, or however we choose to talk about death, we can't avoid it. The reality of our impending death will not change. We will all deal with the death of our loved ones and ourselves in due time.

We can fear the experience or we can embrace it. We can learn how to talk about it, understand it and grow from it. As we and our loved ones approach death, we can claim the remaining moments to talk with them about their death and about the lives we shared. As important as it is to talk about how we live our lives and how to live healthy, balanced and abundant lives, it's also important to talk about end of life.

Talking openly about the issues associated with death and dying helps us alleviate our fears. Communicating with each other about our thoughts and fears can turn death into an experience that enhances our lives—an opportunity not to be wasted. Talking about death creates openness, compassion and empathy, which make our lives better.

For all of us, death is the final curtain call, our last sleep. Death circumscribes our creativity, relationships, experiences and the values we bring to the world, our families and others. Death is the end of all we can do. It is our final experience of life on earth.

> *"Be sure you live your life, because you are a long time dead."*
> — Scottish proverb

Most people in North America die in a hospital. I have seen many deaths during my career as a nurse. I have cared for people who have died quickly and others who have lingered for months. Some have died at peace with themselves and their world, while others have struggled to hold onto their last breath. I have seen the young die and the elderly die. I have seen their families in pain, hurting and crying. I have cried with them. My colleagues and I have shed many a hidden tear and offered up many silent prayers as we were witness to their passing and while we prepared their bodies for transfer to the hospital morgue.

Some have been a source of strength and encouragement to family and friends when they were dying, despite their pain and suffering. They have gone in peace, leaving a sense of hope for others. Some were unprepared and angry about their passing. Perhaps they did not find satisfaction in their lives or they had unresolved conflicts with people in their lives.

We are comfortable talking about birth, sex and politics, but uncomfortable talking about death. We talk openly about many life events and people, about sports, celebrities and vacations. We talk about our children, friends and co-workers. But we do not talk openly about death and dying. Even healthcare professionals find it difficult.

Using the acronym **DEATH**, **D**elivering **E**arth's **A**ngels **T**o **H**eaven, may open us up to engaging in conversations about death with greater comfort. If we visualize our loved ones traveling to a special place, perhaps it would lead us to be more open to talking about it. Others may take comfort from believing in reincarnation or becoming at one with the universe.

I understand many people do not believe in heaven or angels, but by considering death as something worthy of experiencing rather than something to fear, deny or avoid, perhaps we could talk more comfortably about the experience. With a change in attitude, we could become open to talking about the time we enjoyed together. We could speak frankly about our impending loss and grief. Perhaps we would be more open to talk about some of the hurts and challenges we had in our relationships and reconcile these relationships before we regret not doing so.

Raymond Kurzweil, a futurist and author of *The Age of Intelligent Machines*, acknowledges that "a great deal of effort goes into avoiding death. We make extraordinary efforts to delay it and often consider its intrusion a tragic event." He goes on to say that death actually gives meaning and importance to our lives. It gives value to time, as time becomes meaningless when we have too much of it.

Death is the great leveler of life. It doesn't discriminate over color, race, gender, age or social status. Death happens to us all.

Death is almost always sad, and there is no way to deny its pain. But there is no need to deny its existence. By experiencing and acknowledging the painful feelings associated with death, we can open the doors to viewing our lives in their entirety.

Dietrich Bonhoeffer, a German Lutheran pastor, theologian and martyr, said, "As time is the most valuable thing we have, because it is the most irrevocable, the thought of any lost time troubles us whenever we look back." He reminds us not to waste an opportunity to experience all aspects of life. If we do not seize the opportunity to have conversations about death and dying, we may be left feeling as if we have missed an important aspect of life.

> *"It's not the years in your life that count. It's the life in your years."*
>
> — Abraham Lincoln (1809–1865), sixteenth president of the United States

Whether our loved one is dying or we are the loved one who is dying, our grief, pain and sense of loss is better dealt with when we share the experience. Bonhoeffer describes time as "the most valuable thing we have." Why not dedicate time to the learning and fulfillment that comes from open communication and dialogue about our feelings, thoughts and experiences around the end of life?

Experiencing Death

The death and dying experience is accompanied by complex responses. We may feel numb and have a sense of yearning, or protest as we face our own death or that of a loved one. We may feel disorganized, restless, guilty, angry and alone. We may cry a lot. We may feel powerful emotions that cause chaos and confusion.

Elisabeth Kübler-Ross, a Swiss psychiatrist, became a recognized authority on death and dying. In her book *On Death and Dying*, she documents how we react to death and discusses our fear of death. She identifies five stages we go through when we realize we are dying. These stages add to our understanding of why we behave the way we do when we face death. These stages are not absolute. Everyone goes through each one in a different sequence and at a different pace.

We can use Dr. Kübler-Ross's five stages as a flexible guide to give us insight as we seek to understand why we respond as we do when facing death. Ultimately, death is about change. Following are the five stages she identified:

1. Denial: "No, not me." This is a typical reaction when we learn we are terminally ill and will die. Denial helps cushion the impact of the awareness that death is inevitable.

2. Anger: "Why me?" Some of us may resent that others will remain healthy and alive while they will die.

3. Bargaining: "Yes, me, but …" In this stage we accept our upcoming death but start to bargain for more time.

4. Depression: "Yes, me." This is a state of preparatory grief, when we get ready to die. We grow quiet and often do not want visitors.

5. Acceptance: "My time is very close now and it's all right." This final phase is not a happy stage, but neither is it unhappy. It may appear devoid of feelings, but it's not resignation; it's simply acceptance.

In his book *I Don't Know What to Say*, Dr. Robert Buckman wrote, "When a person is dying, his friends and family can no longer deny the reality of death, but if they have not previously acknowledged its existence, they will be ill prepared to face it." When we deny death or avoid talking about it, we create a barrier. We build a wall between those who are dying and their families and friends, isolating them at the very time they most need our support. As a result, the dying person often experiences a social death long before physical death occurs.

When we deny something, in essence, we are saying it does not exist. We are lying to ourselves and others. Living in **DENIAL** of something is another way of saying "I **D**on't **E**ven **N**otice **I A**m **L**ying." Denying the existence of our loved one's terminal illness is like saying "I don't even notice he/she is dying!"

How sad it is to refuse to acknowledge our loved one will be leaving us soon. If they were moving to another community or going on a long trip, we would take time to see them, talk to them and laugh with them. We would take time to say good-bye. Some would host a farewell party.

What a lost opportunity it is when we live in **DENIAL** of the impending death of a family member or friend. What a loss it is when we do not take the time to say, "Good-bye! I so enjoyed having you in my life. I enjoyed the fun, the laughter and the joy of you. I enjoyed the trips, the walks and the conversations. I enjoyed the lessons I learned from you. I truly appreciate the guidance and wisdom you gave me. I know we had times of turmoil and times of conflict, but we worked it out. We learned from it and grew. Thank you for being a part of my life. Thank you for loving me,

"No one ever told me that grief felt so much like fear."

— C.S. Lewis (1898–1963), Irish author and lay theologian

"I'm not that afraid to die. I just don't want to be there when it happens."

— Woody Allen, American director, actor, comedian and author

"Too often we begin to regard a person who is dying as less than living. It is important for us to see each patient as the unique individual that they are right up to the moment of their death."

— David Aaron Kessler, American pediatrician, lawyer and author respecting me and caring for me! I'll always remember you! I love you! I'll miss you! I'll keep you and my cherished memories of you close to my heart."

Why not fill the latter stretches of time we have with our loved ones with a time of understanding, with a time of conversing about the joys and learning we shared together instead of avoiding death's existence. Creating the time for conversations about our shared experiences and discussing the issues surrounding death help us accept the realities of our lives and avoid the potential regrets of those left behind.

> *"Somebody ought to tell us, right at the start of our lives, that we are dying. Then we might live life to the limit every minute of every day."*
>
> — Michael Landon (1936–1991), American actor, writer, director and producer

Just as we have a need to talk with greater ease about the reality of death, we need to talk with greater honesty about the reality of what life is like after the death of our loved ones. Through several studies, George Bonanno, professor of clinical psychology at Columbia University and researcher in the field of grief and trauma, has shown that the bereaved are stronger than they may think.[2] As we accept the death of our loved ones, we are more likely to experience a yearning for them rather than anger or depression because they have died.

> *"We are afraid to live, but scared to die."*
>
> — Inderpal Bahra

In his book *The Other Side of Sadness*, George Bonanno writes that he found widows are more resilient than they are given credit for. He reveals how our inborn emotions of anger, denial, relief and joy help

---

2. Joe Levine, "The New Face of Sadness: George Bonanno Has Redefined Our Thinking about Grief and Resilience," *TC Today* 36, no. 1 (2012), www.tc.columbia.edu/news.htm?articleID=8311&pub=7&issue=280.

us deal effectively with loss. He shows how grieving goes beyond sadness, deepens our connections and can be a positive experience.

Hospice Palliative Care

Hospices and palliative care are for people who are terminally ill—people whose lives and health can no longer be sustained. It is for people who are close to death and are no longer receiving active medical interventions. They receive supportive medical care to alleviate pain and keep them comfortable as they come to the end of their lives. Their families also receive support.

The hospice palliative care movement grew out of the holistic caregiving model for hospice care introduced in England in the 1960s by Dame Cicely Saunders. Dr. Saunders was concerned about the treatment of the dying in hospitals where they were effectively ignored as failures of the medical system. She established the hospice, a place for those who were dying and their families. In the hospice, the individuals with terminal illness could be treated for physical pain and have their psychological, social and spiritual needs met by a team of professionals and volunteers. Their families would be there to support them and, in turn, be supported.

The hospice palliative care concept was brought to North America in 1974. American hospices are not consistently a physical building like the British hospices. They are based on a concept of care that involves teams of medical personnel, professionals and volunteers who assist family caregivers and ensure their dying loved ones have appropriate care and pain management in

> *"You matter because you are you. You matter to the last moment of your life and we will do all that we can, not only to help you die peacefully, but also to live until you die."*
>
> — Dame Cicely Mary Saunders (1918–2005), English nurse, physician, author and founder of St. Christopher's Hospice in Sydenham, England

their own homes. The visiting volunteers are trained to provide companionship, simple comforts and peace of mind to caregivers and family members. The teams also provide bereavement support for those dealing with the death of a loved one.

Hospice palliative care is a valuable resource for those dealing with death and end-of-life issues. It helps people understand and cope as it gives them choices. It does not hasten or delay death, but it comforts and empowers the dying on the final leg of their life's journey. Hospice palliative care offers information, support, hope, dignity, meaning and compassionate care. (Please see appendix III.)

The following poem, written by a child in the Children's Hospice in Minsk, Belarus, sums up what people want to receive at the end of their lives.

When my life is finally measured in
Months, weeks, days, hours,
I want to live free of pain,
Free of indignity, free of loneliness.
Give me your understanding,
Give me your love,
Then let me go peacefully
And help my family to understand.

The following poem has become a popular reading at funerals. It addresses our grief for the loss of a loved one and encourages us to move on, to live and to enjoy our lives.

Remember Me

You can shed tears when I have gone,
but smile instead because I have lived.

Do not shut your eyes and pray to God that I'll come back,
but open your eyes and see all that I have left behind.
I know your heart will be empty because you cannot see me,
but still I want you to be full of the love we shared.
You can turn your back on tomorrow
and live only for yesterday,
or you can be happy for tomorrow because of
what happened between us yesterday.
You can remember me and grieve that I have gone,
or you can cherish my memory and let it live on.
You can cry and lose yourself,
become distraught and turn your back on the world,
Or you can do what I want —
smile, wipe away the tears, learn to
love again and go on.

— David Harkins, English painter and poet

Sustaining Life, Delaying Death

Modern medicine has remarkable powers to prolong life. People with cancer or progressive diseases, accident victims and our frail, elderly parents live longer with the aid of machines and modern medicine. Today, people who would have died live weeks, months, even years longer. For many, this is wonderful. But even though modern medicine and technology can bring us amazing benefits, these interventions also have consequences.

Knowing when to say, "That's enough," "No more" or "Let's pull the plug" has many ramifications. What are the emotional costs to family members when medical intervention is not used to prolong life? What are the physical, emotional and financial costs to families and the healthcare system when life is prolonged? Are costs for sustaining life worth the price we pay? But what are the emotional, physical and financial costs when we don't pay the price? With either option, how do we begin to measure the consequences?

A nineteen-year-old male attends a bush party. He's having fun, enjoying a few drinks around the campfire, laughing and joking with his friends. Someone says something that angers another; a fire log is picked up and swung. The nineteen-year-old is in the line of fire and the log hits his head. He falls to the ground, unresponsive. Someone calls 911, and the young man is rushed to the hospital. Everything is done to save his life. He is attached to a ventilator. In time, his condition stabilizes, he is taken off the ventilator, but brain damage has occurred. For the rest of his life he will be fed by a tube, he will never be able to converse effectively with his family and friends and he will not leave the confines of his hospital bed or chair.

Jackie's ninety-one-year-old mother has just been transferred back to the nursing home where she has lived for the past eight years. Through the aid of active medical interventions, she has survived yet another episode of pneumonia exacerbated by congestive heart failure and other chronic medical conditions. Jackie's mom has not recognized her for over five years; she is fed by the nursing-home staff, has her incontinence pads changed five to six times a day and sits in her wheelchair as the world goes by.

John is sixty-eight years old. He spends most of his days in the hospital. He has type 1 diabetes, which is often out of control. He is on continuous oxygen to help him breath because he has suffered with COPD (chronic obstructive pulmonary disease) for many years. Three times a week he is transported by ambulance from the hospital to the local dialysis unit. There he receives a four-hour hemodialysis treatment, where he is attached to a machine to cleanse and filter his blood to rid his body of harmful wastes. He has a pacemaker implanted under the skin of his chest that sends electrical impulses to his heart muscle to maintain a healthy heart rate and rhythm.

Steve, Martha, Connie, Ben and Bill meet to discuss how to manage their eighty-nine-year-old father's medical condition. He has been admitted to the hospital with his third heart attack. His condition is stabilized and he is recovering well. Since their mother passed away a few years ago, the siblings question whether it is wise for their father to continue living on his own. They question what type of support is available and what quality of life he will have. In collaboration with their father, the doctor asks the family how they want the medical team to respond should his condition worsen. If his heart stops again, do they want the medical team to treat him aggressively by performing CPR and giving him medications and other interventions to sustain his life, or do they prefer to allow nature to take its course?

Dr. Richard Fowler, a critical-care physician at Sunnybrook Hospital in Toronto, said, "I worry that as we have put medicine out there as a potential savior and, in fact, almost a new religion over the last 100 years, people have increasingly bought what we've sold: that cancer can be beaten and every death is a preventable death."[3]

When do we say enough, no more? When do we say we have done all we can? When does quality of life trump medicine, and when do the amazing medical advances we have discovered trump quality of life? Who will approve, give and sign the Do Not Resuscitate order instructing healthcare staff not to revive their patient should their condition worsen or their heart stop? Who will make the decision to change a person's medical status to one of palliative care? Who will say, "Let them die in peace?" I cannot answer these questions for you, but I encourage you and your loved ones to think and talk about how you want to live life and how you want to die.

Dr. Brian Cuthbertson, chief of critical care at Sunnybrook Hospital, said, "When we're talking about whether someone is going to get better, it's not just about will they survive to leave an intensive-care unit, to leave the hospital, but will they have a quality of life that they

3. Lisa Priest, "Critical Care: Spending 10 Weeks with Patients Facing Death," *Globe and Mail* (November 26, 2011), www.theglobeandmail.com/life/health/end-of-life/critical-care-spending-10-weeks-with-patients-facing-death/article2250356/.

want and will accept." He continued, "One of the great challenges of modern medicine is not saying, 'Can we?' but 'Should we?'"[4]

A recent report by the Royal Society of Canada on end-of-life decision making revealed that although competent adults want to be involved in making decisions about their care, most fail to complete advance directives or communicate their preferences to their family and healthcare professionals.[5]

People can make their wishes clear before their family and physicians are forced to make those decisions without them. They can create a living will or advance directives, which they sign, date and have witnessed. The following is one such directive that can be found on the Internet.

> To my family, my physicians, my lawyer and to all others whom it may concern:
>
> Death is as much a reality as birth, growth, maturity and old age; it is the one certainty of life. If the time comes when I can no longer take part in decisions for my own future, let this statement stand as an expression of my wishes and directions, while I am still of sound mind.
>
> If at such time the situation should arise in which there is no reasonable expectation of my recovery from extreme physical and mental disability, I direct that I be allowed to die and not be kept alive by medications, artificial means or "heroic measures." I do, however, ask that medication be mercifully administered to me to alleviate suffering, even though this may shorten my remaining life.

---

4. Ibid.
5. Udo Schuklenk et al., "End-of-Life Decision Making," *Royal Society of Canada Report* (November 2011), www.rsc.ca/documents/RSCEndofLifeReport2011_EN_Formatted_FINAL.pdf.

This statement is made after careful consideration and is in accordance with my strong convictions and beliefs. I want the wishes and directions here expressed carried out to the extent permitted by law. Insofar as they are not legally enforceable, I hope that those to whom this Will is addressed will regard themselves as morally bound by these provisions.[6]

In her article in the *Globe and Mail*, Lisa Priest wrote, "Those who have not given written or explicit verbal directions to relatives may find themselves in critical-care units, unable to stop very aggressive treatments of marginal benefit, as families push for them simply because they feel it's the safest default position."[7]

Talking about and instituting formal advance directives, such as a living will, for yourself and your family members goes a long way to alleviating the difficult decisions that need to be made in regards to sustaining and prolonging life. The choices made today impact you and your family, the medical staff and the healthcare system. They impact how you live out your life and how you will be remembered.

Leaving a Legacy of Your Life

When you know how to live well, you can also learn how to die well. In doing so, you will leave behind a legacy you can be proud of. One that inspires your family, friends and associates.

When you contemplate the impact of your life on this world and consider what is important to you, think about how you

> *"When the time comes to die, make sure that all you have to do is die!"*
> — Elisabeth Elliot, American author and speaker

---

6. Alex Tang, "A Living Will: Samples," *Kairos Spiritual Formation*, www.kairos2.com/a_living_will.htm.

7. Lisa Priest, "Critical Care."

want to be remembered, what your epitaph will say and the example you leave behind.

Remember the story about the dash? The dash is found between the two dates inscribed on a headstone. The dates represent the years lived, but the real story is contained in the dash. Our lives are about how we live, what we accomplish and the impact we have on family, friends, colleagues and the rest of humanity. The dash on our headstones is our legacy. What will your legacy be?

> *"The purpose of life is to be useful, to be honorable. It is to be compassionate. It is to matter, to have it make some difference that you lived."*
>
> Leo C. Rosten (1908–1997), American teacher, academic and humorist

The years before my dad's death were scattered with numerous visits to the doctor and hospital. We lived with the uncertainty of his health and how long his body would sustain him. As a family, we never spoke openly about our father's impending death. However, during those years I often thought about him, his life and how I would feel when he died. I guess you could say I thought about his legacy.

Through his legacy, I came to see my father as an individual, someone who held many roles in his life and who also faced many challenges. He lived a good, full and respectable life. He took risks and he worked hard to provide for the family he loved. He did this within the context of what he knew, using guidelines and values instilled in him through his Dutch Catholic upbringing.

My dad left a first-rate legacy, which was confirmed by the many family members, friends, neighbors, colleagues, church members and acquaintances who came to bid him farewell at his visitation and funeral service. They came to share stories about his life and how he impacted their lives with his humor, compassion and strength. They told us of his generosity and life experiences, some of which we were unaware of and even surprised us. Families are not always aware of the full scope of its members' experiences and character traits. We do not always see our loved ones in the same light as others do.

My father, Gerardus Franciscus VanderDoelen, was born on December 12, 1925, and was raised in a small farming community in Vinkel, Noord-Brabant, the Netherlands. At the age of five, he and his four siblings lost their mother. Shortly after, his father remarried and my dad became a member of a blended family. He lived in occupied Holland during World War II. After the war he became a soldier, fighting guerilla warfare in the then Dutch colony of Indonesia. When he returned three years later, he married my mother and they immigrated to Canada. During his first fifteen years in Canada, he pursued his dream of owning a farm, but, in the end, his dream did not come to fruition. He was an honest man who worked hard and managed his finances well. He provided for his wife and seven children by working full-time during weekdays and part-time in the evenings and on weekends. He was a friend, church member and colleague. He was a son, brother, nephew and an uncle. He was a husband, dad and granddad. He laughed, made jokes and enjoyed playing cards, walking and spending time with family and friends.

I would say he left his wife, children, grandchildren and those whose lives he touched a legacy. He lived his life well. What will your legacy be?

Planning for Your Passing

Making plans for how you live your life is important, but making plans for how you leave your life is also important. In addition to preparing directives regarding end-of-life care, it is important to make plans for the time when you cannot care for yourself and your property and for the effective and efficient distribution of your estate.

This task, which includes preparing a will and keeping it up to date, is overlooked by more than fifty percent of the population. We often hear stories about the controversy and conflicts that arise when a family member becomes ill, is near death and passes away. These stories of family strife and frustration are punctuated with misunderstandings, hurt, jealousy, greed and unresolved issues. They bring stress to everyone involved.

There can be confusion about the rights and responsibilities of those who have been designated as power of attorney over personal care and property. Issues regarding family finances and how they are allocated frequently cause conflicts. Families become divided over money and treasured family possessions, to the point where differences may never be reconciled. Without proper planning and communication, problems arise when children are left with an exorbitant amount of taxes to pay, or when, unknown to family members, the deceased has left a large portion of their assets to a charity. Delays and confusion in how to finalize estate matters can also arise when the family executors are unskilled or have limited knowledge of their responsibilities.

Experienced estate lawyers and trustees are often more efficient and effective in executing the wishes of the deceased. The many problems in settling estates continues to keep our courts and lawyers busy as family members and friends deal with long, expensive and drawn-out processes that could have been avoided. When we plan and communicate our intentions before the time to do so arises, we avoid stress and controversy.

Engaging in actions that will improve future outcomes and ensure all our affairs are in order is **A B**etter **C**hoice. The preparation and planning involved in a well-conceived estate plan will open the door to dialogue surrounding future health issues, estate distribution, charities and death. As you and your family move through the full estate-planning process, you will have numerous opportunities to address concerns and issues.

Planning for your future passing is in your best interest and in the best interest of those you love. It leads to peace of mind as it lays out all your wishes, protects your family and safeguards the assets you have accumulated throughout your lifetime. Planning for the distribution of your estate is healthy for all concerned. A complete estate plan provides those left to finalize your affairs with instruction as to how you wish to have your worldly goods distributed and managed when you die. As you make your plans, consider the best way to

- distribute your assets in accordance to your wishes,

- provide for your loved ones and maximize proceeds to them,

- ensure there are enough funds in your estate to pay for taxes,

- ensure guardianship for your minor children and disabled family members, and

- provide financial support to your favorite charities.

At the same time, work toward avoiding

- needless taxation,

- family strife,

- delays in the settling of your estate,

- costly legal challenges, and

- loss of control of family assets, such as a cottage, a farm, other property or the family business.

Some believe having a will is all they need when planning for the end of their lives, but this is not so. A complete estate plan encompasses many elements, including the following:

- Provide a record of personal papers and information: Keep an inventory of all your assets and liabilities and a list of all your important papers, certificates and documents. Knowing the whereabouts of all your personal information, documents, memberships and subscriptions, as well as the names and contact information for your professional and financial advisors is crucial for your powers of attorney (POA) and executors. Don't forget to list PINs and access codes for all your accounts.

- Prepare a valid will: A will is a legal document, prepared during your lifetime, which takes effect upon your death. It directs the manner in which your executor will distribute your assets and possessions when you die. Because laws change, and because changes occur in families, review your will every five years or every time there is a change in your family situation. Inform a minimum of two people where your will is kept. To ensure objectivity, some prefer to appoint two executors.

  – In *What Was Your Great Grandmother's Name?*, Keith Thomson, a financial educator, consultant and certified financial planner, asks, "What do Michael Jackson, Pablo Picasso, Sonny Bono, Howard Hughes, Jimi Hendrix, and Abraham Lincoln have in common?" He answers, "They all died without a will." One out of every two Canadians dies *intestate*; they die without a will. If you do not have a will, the government decides how your assets will be distributed.

- Plan for incapacity: Prepare a Power of Attorney (POA) form for personal care and for property. This document legally defines the individual(s) who will act on your behalf while you are alive but no longer able to make decisions about your personal care or property. This eliminates the need for a court-appointed administrator who does not know you. Normally the POA document will also provide a living will or advance directives on the way in which you wish your end-of-life affairs to be dealt with.

- Plan for reducing taxes and probate fees: A key objective in estate planning is to reduce or postpone taxes that are payable at your death. Talk with your financial advisor to learn how to reduce probate fees and taxes at the time of your death, as there are various ways to do this, and maximize the assets you bequeath to others.

- Preplan your funeral: Making your own funeral arrangements relieves loved ones of additional stress when you die. Family members and/or funeral homes can help sort out the details and the costs with you.

- Plan to donate your organs: The need for organs and tissues continues to outweigh availability, and giving someone a second chance to live is a great legacy to leave behind. Organs and tissues that may be donated include the heart, liver, kidneys, pancreas, lungs, small bowel, stomach, corneas, heart valves, bone and skin. A donor's eligibility is determined by the healthcare team upon death. (Please see appendix III.)

Giving to Others

Any form of giving is *philanthropy*. Many people associate philanthropy with money, but it is defined as "the effort or inclination to increase the well-being of humankind." It means "love of mankind," coming from the Greek words *philien*, "to love," and *anthropos*, "mankind."

We can give our time, talents and/or treasures. Giving brings joy to the giver and the receiver. It helps make the world a better place and gives many a purpose for living. Giving to others creates part of our legacy. Giving at the time of our passing enhances our legacy. It's often the time in which we can offer our most significant contribution to the causes that are dear to our hearts.

Giving is a very personal and individual matter. A British article highlighted the various reasons we have for giving to charity:

- To feel good about ourselves

- A reaction to a life experience—a birth, death, disaster or tragedy

- To promote our self-image

- Growing up in a charitable environment

> *"The more you give, the more you have. Abundance creates the ability to give; giving creates more abundance."*
>
> — Jim Stovall, American author and speaker

- A way to give back and say thank you[8]

Giving helps us make the world a better place. Our financial gifts feed our communities' hungry, shelter the homeless, heal the sick, educate children, sustain the arts, care for the elderly, mentor youth, house stray animals and maintain a healthy ecosystem.

Giving can create a sense of satisfaction that comes with knowing that we are helping others. People who give are happier than those who do not. Giving is good for the giver and the receiver as it draws on our need to connect, to be positive and to be involved in something good.

You Don't Need to Be Rich to Give

In 2000, I began to transition from nursing to a career in fundraising. As a professional fundraiser, I was able to enjoy the company of many generous supporters of the organizations I worked for. Many had wonderful stories to share about their lives and their giving, but my biggest philanthropic hero is an elderly retiree who gave out of complete commitment and love.

Gladys did not give a large sum to our organization, but she gave every year, which means a lot to a charity. One day I went to her home to express our appreciation. When I arrived, I knew her capacity to give would never be large. Three sets of locks had to be unbolted before she could let me into her bachelor apartment. Gladys told me that when she first moved into the building it was a seniors' residence, but the government had changed the building to low-income housing some years back. Living in the building today meant Gladys

---

8. Alan Cole, "Overview: Charity Giving," *Xperedon Charity News* (August 11, 2011), www.xperedon.com/news_659.

frequently heard gun shots, witnessed fights and smelled the odor of drugs.

Gladys informed me that she had been a waitress all her life, starting in Newfoundland at age fifteen. She shared that she raised her three children on her own and was therefore never able to give them very much. Today she lives on her Canada and Old Age Security pensions.

When I asked why she supported the organization I represented, and who else she supported, she said, "I give to sixty different organizations. I enjoy giving. It makes me feel good."

Gladys gave each organization $15 a year and would not think of taking any of them off her list. "They're all important to me," she said. Her funds supported children, locally and abroad. They supported health-related organizations, education, the environment and animals. She gave approximately eight percent of her small income each year to charity. When she filed her income tax return, she applied for the charitable tax credits and received a refund, which she then gave to her three children. They encouraged her to keep the money for herself, but she told them she hadn't been able to give them much when they were little, so she wanted to give them what she could now.

To me, that's a story of loving generosity, a story of philanthropy and an outstanding legacy story. When I think of what and how Gladys gave back to others, I am in awe and my heart goes out to her.

My primary focus as a fundraiser was on creating awareness and educating others on how to give at their passing. In the profession, this is known as Planned Giving or Legacy Giving.

When I met with supporters of charitable organizations, we spoke about their lives and experiences. They shared with me

> *"Do all the good you can, by all the means you can, in all the ways you can, in all the places you can, at all the times you can, to all the people you can, as long as you can."*
>
> — John Wesley (1703–1791), English clergyman and theologian

why they gave to the organization I represented and to other organizations. I shared aspects about the organization and introduced giving opportunities they could incorporate into their estate plans. They became aware of ways to continue to offer support to the charities they cared for after they passed away. This gave them the potential to decrease their estate taxes and probate fees and increase what they gave their families and favorite causes.

Many who give of their time, talent and treasure to a cause during their lifetimes do not do so in their passing. Over eighty percent of Canadians give financial support to charities, but only seven percent of the population gives to charity in their passing. And that seven percent applies only to those who had drawn up a will.[9]

> *"As good stewards we must think carefully about our assets, invest them wisely, and pray for guidance about how to give them away."*
>
> — The United Church of Canada, *Will Workbook*

My husband, a chartered accountant, managed the accounts of a church for many years. It was a church where people would often practice tithing, the giving of ten percent of one's income. When I asked if the church ever received a gift through someone's will, he said no. People who give financially throughout their lifetimes often do not give in their passing because no one asked them, and they are seldom aware of the benefits it can provide to their children and charitable organizations.

A study in 2008 showed that those who leave a charitable gift in their will live three years longer than those who don't.[10]

Many believe that by giving a gift to charity in their will, they are disinheriting their children, but this is not true. In his previously mentioned book, Keith Thomson explains, "With the implementation

---

9. Canadian Association of Gift Planners, "Statistics on Giving" (2012), www.leavealegacy.ca/program/who.

10. Ibid.

of a number of fairly straightforward financial planning techniques, you can choose to redirect your tax dollars in such a manner that your estate pays no tax and your favorite philanthropic organization receives the financial benefit. Ultimately, as a result of this kind of tax planning, your children could actually end up with more! Think of it this way, giving through your estate could be thought of as adopting another child … while disinheriting the taxman."

Michael Posner, a writer for Toronto's *Globe and Mail*, interviewed Peter Munk, founder and chairman of Barrick Gold Corporation. He asked him if his children will receive his wealth when he dies. Peter Munk explained, "I love my five children, but other causes are more worthy. My wealth will do more good for a hospital than a bigger car for my daughter." He said that he believes in giving everything away, that the money belongs to society. He said that his children "will get an excellent education and an understanding that life is about integrity and not compromising your values; that it's about what you contribute, not what you take out."[11]

Giving a legacy gift is not just for the wealthy. During my fundraising career, I found the largest gifts came from average, everyday people. Consider how these ordinary people made extraordinary differences in the lives of others when they incorporated legacy giving into their estate plans:

- Eleanor and thirty friends celebrated a tugboat launch at a lake near her home. The day honored the friendship and vibrancy of sixty-three-year-old Eleanor, who had built a replica of a Harbor tug in her garage. Just three months later, she died of cancer and her friends gathered with her again. Eleanor's ability to persevere through the challenges of her disease lives on in her legacy gift. In leaving a gift in her will to fund cancer

---

11. Michael Posner, "Peter Munk's Reflections on Being a Winner," *CTV News Online* (2011), www.ctv.ca/generic/generated/static/business/article1913769. html.

research, she knew that if one small woman could build a tugboat, a future without cancer could happen.

- – The most common type of legacy gift is a gift or bequest made in your will. A gift in your will can be a specific amount, a percentage or a residual amount, or it can be your entire estate. In Canada, charitable receipts can be claimed in one's final tax return, up to 100 percent of net income in the year of death.

- When Peter told his family he had a life-threatening disease, he asked, "What positive can we learn from the experience?" His positive message is building a healthier future for others with the gift he gave when he made his local hospital the beneficiary of his life insurance policy.

  - – When a charity is named as full or partial beneficiary of a new or existing life insurance policy, your estate receives a charitable tax receipt for the value received from the policy. Gifts of life insurance are exempt from probate fees, and unlike a gift in your will, they remain private and confidential.

- Lynn was walking home from the grocery store. As she crossed the street, she was hit by a car and suffered major injuries and brain damage. As she lay in an intensive-care bed, Lynn's family informed the healthcare team that she had signed an organ donation card. Her organs improved and saved the lives of those waiting for organ transplants. Lynn's legacy lives on in the lives of others. It also lives on in the work of others because she named her local community foundation as the beneficiary of her retirement funds.

  - – Many people have significant assets in their retirement funds (RRSPs and RRIFs). Naming a spouse as the designated beneficiary of these plans defers the tax liability. If the sur- viving spouse were to designate a charity as a full or partial beneficiary of these retirement funds, their estate receives a charitable tax receipt for the full value of this gift. The tax credit from the gift may lower income taxes payable at death. Gifts of retirement funds also remain private and confidential and are exempt from probate fees.

- John was a community builder and industry leader. When he died, his leadership continued. Through a gift of securities, he set up an endowment fund at his local university. As in life, others follow his lead. Yearly, family and friends boost John's fund with gifts made in his honor.

  - When stocks and securities that have appreciated are sold, fifty percent of the capital gains must be reported as income. By donating them to charity (either while you are living or at the time of your death), the charity receives the full market value of the shares and your estate receives a charitable tax receipt for their full value. When you give in this way, all the capital gains are eliminated and you pay no tax. (Note: The capital gains exemption is lost if you sell the shares first and then donate the cash to charity.)

These four methods of legacy giving, through a gift (1) in your will, (2) of life insurance, (3) of retirement funds or (4) of securities, are simple to arrange. A knowledgeable financial advisor can assist you. Remember to inform your family and the charity of your intentions. (Please see appendix III.)

The Charity Child

Knowing I worked in the charitable sector, people often said, "I wish I had money that I could give away, but I don't have the big bucks like Bill Gates or Warren Buffet. I'm not sure if I'll have enough to take me through the retirement years, and I don't want to become a financial burden to my children or anyone else."

I would respond, "Well, you're not alone. I think we all wish we had more to give away to help others. However, something you might like to think about for the future is having a charity child in your will."

"A charity child! What's that?"

I explained, "Well, the next time you update your will, think about dividing your estate like an apple pie. Say you have two children and some friends or family you want to include in your will. Divide the pie into sections and leave the last piece for your favorite charity. It's good for you and for the charity, and it will help with estate taxes. You'll be leaving a little legacy on earth for future generations."

People understand this when it's explained to them. I can see the wheels turning as they begin to imagine an apple pie and the portion sizes of who would get what. It's easy to understand and put into action.

To understand and learn more about the benefits and the how-tos of this type of giving, speak with an experienced financial advisor.

> *"Taxes are our way of feeding the goose that lays the golden eggs of freedom, democracy, and enterprise. Someone says, 'Well, the goose eats too much.' That's probably true. But better a fat goose than no goose at all!"*
>
> — Jim Rohn (1930–2009), American entrepreneur, author and motivational speaker

Giving to the Government While Cutting Your Tax Bill

My writings on giving included several ways to maximize the net-of-tax money we have left to bequeath to our families and to the greater good. Minimizing our tax bills is important as we build our financial health, but we also need to appreciate how taxes play an important role in our society. They give us benefits and privileges we would be unable to enjoy otherwise. By paying our taxes, we support and sustain a lifestyle that provides us with

- well-kept streets, roads and sidewalks, enabling us to enjoy ease in moving about;

- police officers patrolling the streets, keeping us safe and giving us the freedom to go shopping or walking about without fear;

- federal, provincial, state, city and town governments to keep us working together in an orderly fashion;

- parks and recreation centers, emergency services and a host of other services that are continually functioning and available to us;

- schools and teachers to educate our children;

- healthcare for when we and our loved ones become ill; and

- a country kept safe by a military equipped and trained to protect us from those who could harm us.

That being said, many begrudge paying taxes. It is possible the word *tax* conjures up images of the taxman, be it the CRA (Canada Revenue Agency) or Uncle Sam (IRS), with their hands in our pockets, grabbing the coins we have diligently worked for and saved.

Canada is one of the highest-taxed nations in the world. Its residents pay almost half their yearly income to taxes, representing a major obstacle in accumulating wealth. In Canada, "Tax Freedom Day" in 2011 was June 6, the day when Canadians, as a nation, had paid all their taxes that year—157 days. It took US residents 102 days, until April 12, to pay their taxes.

While the government is diligent in collecting taxes from us, tax legislation also provides socially responsible ways to minimize the transition of money from our pockets to theirs. When building financial health, it is wise to implement effective tax-saving strategies to maximize the wealth we accumulate and the money we have available to sustain our needs and desires. Following are **TIP**s **T**o **I**mprove your **P**erformance in minimizing our tax liabilities:

- Registered retirement savings plans: Registered retirement funds offer substantial tax deductions.

- Donations: Charitable donations allow Canadians personal tax credits worth up to forty-six percent.

- Education: Depending on the educational institution you attend and if your course is post-secondary, vocational or job related, you may be able to qualify for a tuition deduction from your taxable income.

- Healthcare plans: In Canada, most medical expenses, including dental work, prescription drugs and nonconventional health practitioners, are tax deductible if they are not covered by an employer-provided health plan.

- Starting an investment portfolio: Certain investment vehicles are taxed at lower rates than ordinary investment income that is earned on bank accounts, bonds, Guaranteed Investment Certificates and the like.

- Starting a business: Business ownership, either your own, a franchise or a home-based business, offers tax-saving opportunities, but the pursuit needs to be balanced against its challenges.

When it comes to tax laws and good money management, make sure you do your research and seek professional advice. Look for assistance to manage risk areas and fill in your knowledge gaps. Tax legislation is complicated and changes frequently, so it is difficult to know all the laws. Be wise and search for a financial advisor who meets your needs, understands your situation and can give you an assessment, recommendations and an action plan.

Embracing Health, Balance and Abundance as You Prepare for Death and Taxes

Death and taxes are inevitable. Both can be unpleasant to deal with. When you are aware of the many issues that encompass death and taxes, you begin to take actions to enhance both experiences. By talking about **DEATH** and dying, you may find the experience adds a new dimension to your life.

Incorporating effective tax strategies into your financial planning will improve your **KASH** flow, now and for the future. Adding effective tax strategies into your estate plans leaves the world a better place and builds a legacy.

It is much easier to improve your life and the world when you have the **K**nowledge, **A**bilities, **S**kills and **H**abits you need to live well, and to die well. Knowing how to make wise decisions regarding your death and the death of your loved ones and how to effectively distribute your estate assets starts when you say …

Let It Begin with Me!

Chapter 9

FUN

What Is FUN?

SpongeBob, the main character in the children's animated television series *SpongeBob SquarePants*, sings a song about **FUN**:

- **F** is for friends who do stuff together,
- **U** is for you and me, and
- **N** is for anywhere and anytime at all.

> *"There ain't much fun in medicine, but there's a heck of a lot of medicine in fun."*
>
> — Josh Billings (1818–1885), American humorist and lecturer

Erik Carlson, a sought-after international speaker, author and life coach explains **FUN** as

- **F**inding your greatness,
- **U**plifting others, and
- '**N**joying the journey.

SpongeBob sings about the fun we have with our friends, whereas Carlson, a member of the International Brotherhood of Magicians, uses inspirational and imaginative presentations about **FUN** to improve people's productivity, service, teamwork and leadership abilities. He encourages people to put **FUN** and **MAGIC** into their lives to **M**ake **A G**reat **I**mpacting **C**hange.

Volkswagen, the car company, has created an initiative called *The Fun Theory*. Their website of the same name is dedicated to the thought that something as simple as fun is the easiest way to change people's behavior for the better.

Fun is enjoyment, amusement or lighthearted pleasure. It's when we are comfortable in our own skin. Fun makes us happy.

The definition of fun is hard to pin down because, essentially, it's subjective. What's fun for one person might be agony for another. Even though the pursuit of knowledge involves hard work, some find studying and learning to be fun. Whatever fun is to us, we know when we're having fun and when we're not.

Many of us think of fun as being pure enjoyment and pleasure. It does not require work or sacrifice. We can go out with friends, read a good book or go to a movie. We do not have to put effort into it, other than simply being there.

Some consider fun to be synonymous with play. Play, like fun, is what we engage in for enjoyment and pleasure and to amuse ourselves. But unlike some types of fun, play is for recreation rather than a serious or practical purpose.

Play is for everyone. We engage in play throughout our lives. Children play every day. Babies play as they explore their hands and feet and the world around them. Young children play when they dress up and pretend. As children become older, they play games and enjoy specific activities and hobbies. We continue to play as we become adults.

Play is a learning experience and can be divided into free and structured play. Free play occurs when we lead the experience and don't set rules and boundaries. We can become engrossed in the activity because we develop it ourselves. Structured play, which is planned, guided and led, can limit and minimize our opportunity to be creative and inventive.

Good-quality play provides activities to stimulate our emotional, physical and intellectual development. It stimulates us imaginatively, constructively, creatively and physically.

- Imaginative play is pretending and fantasy, which develops self-expression and our ability to see things from other people's points of view. It develops our social skills.

- Constructive play is a process of building an end product from a range of materials. It promotes our motor skills and encourages language skills when we talk about what we are doing.

- Creative play ranges from arts and crafts to music and dance. It gives us the opportunity to develop fine manipulative skills.

- Physical play covers many indoor and outdoor activities. It can involve equipment or not, and it develops fine and gross motor skills, along with muscle control. It encourages healthful living habits and results in better eating and sleeping habits. It develops self-confidence and physical competencies.

Play is often described as the *work* of childhood. It is a vital part of our children's holistic development. Through play, children explore their world, take risks, make mistakes and achieve. Through play, they

> *"Play is a fun, enjoyable activity that elevates our spirits and brightens our outlook on life. It expands self-expression, self-knowledge, self-actualization and self-efficacy. Play relieves feelings of stress and boredom, connects us to people in a positive way, stimulates creative thinking and exploration, regulates our emotions and boosts our ego."*
>
> — Garry Landreth, American psychologist and author

learn to use their imaginations and develop creative thinking; they learn to express themselves. It is through play that we build relationships with each other and those who play alongside us. It offers us choice, control and freedom within reasonable boundaries.

We continue to need play as adults. It enhances our social interactions and our cognitive ability to learn new skills. Those of us who do not take part in play are more likely to suffer the impact of stress. We may experience boredom and depression. To minimize our stress level and improve our happiness quotient, it is important for us to have at least one activity that we do regularly just for fun.

Hobbies and other fun activities provide us with entertaining ways to sharpen our skills, express our creativity or blow off steam. When we are able to fully engross ourselves in an activity we enjoy, we can experience a state of being in which our brains are in a near-meditative state, benefitting our bodies, minds and souls.

Many hobbyists find their interests to be a continual source of relaxation and stress relief. Some have turned their hobbies into careers, giving them a lifestyle in which their work is their play.

The saying "All work and no play make Jack a dull boy" holds more truth than most realize. Research indicates that without play, it is hard to give our best at work or at home. The healing powers of play are coming to be appreciated more as psychotherapists learn and use various approaches and techniques to integrate play into their practices.

The National Institute of Play says play is the gateway to vitality, and that by its very nature, play is uniquely and intrinsically rewarding and healing. It generates optimism, seeks out novelty and makes perseverance fun as it leads to mastery. It gives the immune system a boost, fosters empathy and promotes a sense of belonging and community. Not engaging in play can lead to health problems and fragility.

Play is good for our relationships. The National Institute of Play says it refreshes long-term adult-adult relationships by bringing humor, the enjoyment of novelty, the capacity to share a lighthearted sense of the world's ironies, the enjoyment of mutual storytelling and the capacity to openly divulge our imaginations and fantasies. Playful communication and interaction produce an atmosphere for easy connection, leading to the deepening of relationships.

Whatever your understanding and interpretation of fun and play is, having it definitely makes life more enjoyable.

What do you do regularly for fun and play? When was the last time you went down a slide, played hide-and-seek or had a good game of ball? You are never too old to play. Play keeps us young and healthier. When we live life without play, we increase our risk of stress-related diseases, mental health problems, addiction and violence.

"Just as children need play to help them de-stress, adults need play to help them be at their best when it comes to career, parenting and marriage. Consider fun and play to be great investments in your well-being."

— Adam Blatner, American psychiatrist, trainer and author

It's a Laughing Matter

We all need to make time to be less serious about life. Smiling at some of the things we do, or just laughing at ourselves, is a way to do this. American actress Ethel Barrymore said, "We grow up the day we have the first real laugh at ourselves."

Q: When is a car not a car?
A: When it turns into a garage.

Q: How much do pirates pay for their earrings?
A: A Buccaneer!

Q: Why did the scientist install a knocker on his door?
A: He wanted to win the No-bell Prize.

Q: Why did the atoms cross the road?
A: It was time to split!

When was the last time you were told by a medical professional to stay home from work and find ways to get yourself laughing, whether it be watching *Seinfeld* or another funny program on TV, going to the circus or laughing with children? Has anyone in the healthcare system said to you, "Tell me about the last time you had a good laugh"?

Laughter is a great way to relieve stress. It helps people cope, be more creative and eliminate boundaries. It makes hard things easier, while helping to prevent mental and physical damage.

Reading a comic, hearing a joke or going to a funny show brings laughter and lightens our lives. When we laugh, our brains release endorphins, which ease pain, increase alertness and make us feel joyful. Laughter and humor diffuse tense situations and relax us.

Laughter is like internal jogging. It enhances respiration and circulation, oxygenates the blood and suppresses the stress-related hormones in the brain. Laughter activates the immune system. It is a powerful antidote to stress.

Laughter releases energy and makes us feel positive. When we laugh at a funny movie or with family or friends, we feel the weight of responsibility lift from our shoulders and slip away.

When was the last time you **LOL**, or **L**aughed **O**ut **L**oud? When you feel tension building, think of how long it has been since you had a good laugh. It may be longer than you realize. The first few lines of the poem "The Laughing Classroom Oath" by Diana Loomans and Karen Kolberg say, "I do solemnly swear from this day forward / to grease my giggling gears each day / and to wear a grin on my face for no reason at all!"

We must balance work and pleasure, giving and receiving and seriousness and levity to assure a contented and healthy life. Just as a car needs refilling with gas or a fridge needs restocking, we need to restore ourselves. If we don't take time to recharge our batteries with fun, play and laughter, we experience negative emotions such as discouragement, depression, despair, anger, resentment and self-pity.

Some people find it difficult to laugh, have fun and play. Life and its burdens drag them down; worry, anxiety and depression take the fun out of their lives. Sometimes people respond to life in unhealthful ways. Their attitude is negative and they try to hide from life. Then there are times, in responding to life's challenges, when we react, or are expected to react, in ways that are against our values and principles, leading to inner turmoil. Feelings of inner turmoil or injustice affect our ability to have fun.

In this chapter I discuss issues that inhibit our ability to have fun. Engaging in activities against our principles and values, working too much and hiding our secrets can limit our ability to have fun. When we have difficulty letting go of issues from the past, we find it hard to relax. Without fun, play and laughter in our lives, our balance wheels of health and well-being may develop a leak.

Principles and Values to Live By

Life principles are the guidelines that keep us accountable and mold our actions. Acting against our principles causes discomfort, turmoil and stress, decreasing the amount of fun we enjoy. Knowing and living by our principles and values enhance our lives.

Remember "The Fisherman" story in the chapter on finance? Both the Mexican and the businessman enjoy a full life. They enjoy time with family and friends, rest and relaxation, the benefits of being an entrepreneur and working. They both live by their values and principles, but they chose different paths.

"People who live based on principles achieve what they desire, while people who live reacting to circumstances do not."

— Chris Widener, American author, leadership coach and speaker

Our values shape us. They represent who we are and what we stand for. We are governed by our values, which influence our decisions and determine how effectively we manage our lives. Values can be instilled in us or we can adopt them. Our values can also change, but it's important to know that when we have strong, positive values, they become an integral part of our achieving what we want in life.

Once we know our values, we can set out to achieve our goals. Many find goal-setting and reaching their goals to be fun. Goals are more specific and personal and are different from our values. Goals refer to set targets, whereas values are universal in character and apply to society as a whole. Goals are the objectives we strive to achieve.

The following chart illustrates how values and goals differ:

| The Differences between Values and Goals ||
Values	Goals
Honesty	Retire at fifty-five
Humility	Stop worrying
Peace of mind	Ski with friends
Integrity	Spend more time with children
Freedom	Go back to school
Courage	Start a business
Family	Learn to paint
Charity	Take a trip to Africa
Spirituality	Lose weight
Education	Give to the sick and poor
Health	Buy a house
Love	Find a supportive partner

Knowing our values makes it easier to formulate our goals and reach our potential. But achieving our goals does not just happen.

Achieving our goals takes action directed by plans. Remember, *if we fail to plan we plan to fail.*

A research study on goal-setting by Gail Matthews and Steven Kraus at Dominican University in California showed that people who write down goals increase the likelihood of achieving them.[1]

A **SMART** guide for planning and writing our goals is to assure that they are

- **S**pecific: Fuzzy targets are too hard to hit.

- **M**easurable: Goals that are hard to measure are hard to achieve.

- **A**ttainable: Make sure the goal itself is reachable.

- **R**ealistic: Consider your personal, physical and financial abilities.

- **T**imely: Create timelines by which to accomplish your goals.

You could say that **SMART** goals are driven by smart principles and values as they create a solid foundation for living life—for our actions and behaviors. The First Nations, Métis and Inuit peoples of North America have seven sacred values, or laws, that are foundational to how they live. Consider incorporating them into your set of values.

1. Love: Always act in love; love the creator, the earth, yourself, your family and your fellow human beings.

2. Respect: Respect all life on earth and your leaders and people of all races.

3. Courage: Listen to your heart and know it takes courage to do what is right.

4. Honesty: Never lie or gossip, be honest with yourself and others and speak from your heart and be true to your word.

---

1. "Do Written Goals Really Make a Difference?" *UGM Consulting* (August 26, 2011), www.ugmconsulting.com/Do%20written%20goals%20really%20 make%20a%20difference%20UGM%20Briefing%2026%20Aug%202011.pdf.

5. Wisdom: Show wisdom in your actions and words and in building a peaceful world.

6. Humility: Think of others before yourself and be humble and thankful.

7. Truth: Always seek truth; living the truth is living by the seven laws.

Having the Right Attitude

Enjoyment and fun come when we have the right attitude, and the right attitude comes from the right focus. When we train our minds to focus on the good rather than the bad, we can take pleasure and satisfaction in what we have and what we are doing.

Our attitudes are affected by our opinions and thoughts. Positive thoughts and opinions produce positive attitudes. Negative thoughts and opinions produce negative attitudes. Positive attitudes fill our lives with good, whereas negative attitudes fill our lives with fear and regret.

One person may look at life and see goodness, beauty, friendship and warmth, whereas another in similar circumstances sees ugliness, loneliness, problems and hopelessness. What makes the difference? Attitude! Our attitudes determine whether we are happy or sad, serene or angry, have fun or live in misery.

Medical research has shown that our bodies produce natural morphine-like substances that operate on specific receptor sites in the brain and spinal cord. These natural opiates are called *endorphins*. Secreted and used by the brain, endorphins reduce the experience of pain and screen out unpleasant stimuli. The presence of endorphins causes feelings of well-being and optimism, while inhibiting feelings of depression.

Behavioral researchers have learned that we can actually stimulate the production of endorphins through optimistic thoughts and a positive attitude. Positive attitudes are like nourishment to the body and soul. Negative thoughts and attitudes deprive the body of endorphins, which leads to depression and more negative thinking. Further, negative attitudes, such as bitterness, anger, blame, mean-spiritedness, revengefulness and ungratefulness, are stressful, leading to hypertension, elevated heart rate, headaches and hormonal imbalances. When we focus our thoughts and conversations on our problems, disappointments and struggles, we fall into the trap of talking negatively. The more we think and talk negatively, the weaker we become.

In *The Power of Positive Thinking*, Norman Vincent Peale explained that when we believe something can be accomplished, and then devote our thoughts, ideas, talents and hard work to it, we can make it happen. When we think something cannot be done, our negative thinking

> **"Change your thoughts and you change your world."**
> — Norman Vincent Peale (1898–1993), American minister and author

affects our abilities and the way we work, and proves it so. The person who consistently has a positive attitude always outperforms the negative thinker.

When we believe that something can be achieved, we release all of our creative energy toward finding solutions to make it happen. If setbacks, challenges or discouragement come our way, as they always do, positive thinking keeps us on track and encourages us to put our best efforts forward.

Complaining, griping, envy, jealousy, pessimism and other negative attitudes, habits or compulsions keep us locked in a dark world. To have more fun and live a better life, these traits need to be removed, but they cannot be rooted out without leaving a vacuum that can suck a person right back into their habitual pattern.

> **"If you don't like something, change it. If you can't change it, change your attitude."**
> — Maya Angelou, American author and poet

Bad attitudes, habits and traits must be replaced with their opposite. "I will" needs to replace "I won't." "I can do it" needs to replace "I can't do it." If we are discontented, we need to cultivate happy thoughts. If we are critical, we need to focus on the good, learn to be thankful and praise others. We need to replace doubts and fears with faith and confidence, and boredom with new habits, actions and skills.

Other **TIP**s to improve your attitude include

> *"Sow a thought and you reap an action; sow an action and you reap a habit; sow a habit and you reap a character; sow a character and you reap a destiny."*
>
> — Ralph Waldo Emerson (1883–1882), American essayist, lecturer and poet

- getting a "checkup" on your attitude and thinking;

- practicing being positive in every situation, especially in the face of adversity;

- developing a positive view of the future;

- examining your attitude daily and guarding it with diligence;

- knowing that your life is as good as you think it to be; and

- remembering that improving your attitude and state of mind takes time.

In This World You Will Have Trouble!

Clearly, a positive attitude is critical to healthy outcomes, but unrealistic expectations can result in disappointment and resentment. Life comes with challenges. It comes with difficulties and problems. Life is not always fair. We all encounter some turmoil in our lives. Behind every face there is a story. Knowing that trials and tribulations are a fact of life protects us from having our peace of mind or personal power stolen from us when they come our way.

In life, as in exercise, when we do more than we think we can and go beyond our comfort zones by pushing ourselves, we build endurance, strength and character. In an exercise routine, we gain ninety percent of our muscle growth when we push ourselves to complete the last two of ten repetitions. Effortless living is not effective living. As with physical exercise, there is no gain without the pain. Instead of resisting life's challenges, consider them to be the training that builds us up.

When you find yourself in a time of trial, you may feel as through you are in the middle of an ocean with a storm raging around you. Do not jump overboard. Instead, learn to stay the course, keep your thoughts and conversations focused on where you are going and respond accordingly. Know that all storms will pass. Do not waver in the direction you set for yourself. Keep moving forward. Don't quit.

Sometimes our troubles reveal an area of our lives that needs to be cleaned up or improved on. Never lose the opportunity to become a better person, spouse, parent, friend, employee, employer or community member. Ask yourself, "What lesson can I learn from this?"

A baby bird must struggle to emerge from its shell. If someone helps it out, the bird will be weak and unable to deal with

> *"Things don't go wrong and break your heart so you can become bitter and give up. They happen to break you down and build you up so you can be all that you were intended to be."*
>
> — Samuel Johnson (1709–1784), British writer and lexicographer

> *"Suffering is the tuition one pays for a character degree. People can use their suffering either to gain character or become bitter. The ones who choose bitterness live a long, slow death. The ones who choose character truly live."*
>
> — Richard M. Rayner, American medical practitioner

"One of the secrets of success is to refuse to let temporary setbacks defeat us."

— Mary Kay Ash (1918–2001), American businesswoman

"Everything has its wonders, even darkness and silence, and I learn whatever state I may be in, therein to be content."

— Helen Keller (1880–1968) American author, activist and first deaf-blind person to earn a BA degree

its environment. However, when we allow it to develop, grow and learn, it will soon be strong enough to stretch its wings and fly. Like the bird, when we struggle with setbacks and challenges, we become stronger and better able to manage and deal with more complex challenges.

Pain in life is inevitable, but suffering is optional. When we learn to accept that trials and tribulations are a part of life, we are better able to endure the difficult times. Roses have thorns. We can't expect to enjoy life's color, beauty and fragrance without accepting that thorny challenges come.

Stop and Rest for a While

In a lecture about stress management, the instructor raised a glass of water and asked, "How heavy is this glass of water?" Answers from the audience ranged from 1 ounce to 8 ounces.

The instructor replied, "The weight doesn't matter. What matters is how long you try to hold it. If you hold it for a minute, it won't be a problem. If you hold it for an hour, your arm will ache. If you hold it for a day, someone will have to call an ambulance for you. In each case the weight is the same, but the longer you hold it, the heavier it becomes."

He continued, "And that is the way it is with stress. If you carry your burdens with you all the time, they will get increasingly heavier, and sooner or later you won't be able to carry on."

Rest and relaxation separate us from the business of life. Taking time to **REST** allows us the time to stop, think and regroup. It gives us time to reflect, adjust and reconsider what is happening in our lives, what may be holding us back and what we can do. During challenging times, take time to **REST** and

- **R**emember how you adjusted and recovered before,
- **E**ntrust you will adjust and be effectively active again,
- **S**tand firm against negative thoughts and actions, and
- **T**ake the lessons from the moment to learn and grow.

When we do not take time for rest and relaxation, we become tired and frustrated. Taking time to refresh ourselves prevents burnout, stress and weariness. Taking time to rest and relax gives us time for fun, play and laughter.

> *"Take rest; a field that has rested gives a beautiful crop."*
> — Ovid (43 BCE– c. CE 17), Roman poet

Excuses

Many of us may prefer to engage in activities we *wanna* do, not *must* do. We do not want to be told what to do or be disciplined. We do not realize that self-discipline is important and valuable in building a healthy, balanced and abundant life. Nor do we realize that *self-discipline's most valuable by-product is self-worth*, which, in turn, impacts our enjoyment of life.

When we are not disciplined, a small infection, if not taken care of, becomes a disease that leads to a loss of self-worth, self-esteem and self-respect. One of life's great temptations is to ease up a little. Instead of seeing our commitments through to fruition, we allow ourselves to quit before the job is done, or we do a little less than our best.

A scientist I know, who originally came from Belgium, was asked to present her research projects to a large audience at an upcoming conference. She was nervous about her strong Belgian accent, as well as her presentation and speaking skills. She said to herself, "I can learn to speak and present better, or I can stay in this laboratory for the rest of my life." Her choice was to discipline herself and obtain new skills. She attended weekly Toastmasters meetings, prepared speeches, took on various roles and completed her Toastmasters' Competent Communicator designation. She now credits her advanced speaking skills as a key factor in securing her dream job, a position as professor at a Belgian university in her home community close to her family and friends.

"I can't," "It's going to cost too much," "I'm not smart enough" and "My health is not good" are all symptoms of the disease called *excusitis.*

Excuses are a way to justify why we haven't accomplished what we said we would. Overcoming and stopping our tendency to make excuses or blame other people and circumstances for our shortfalls are better choices for living a better life. Telling people how we accomplished our success is much more uplifting and fun than telling them why we didn't. Making excuses or playing the blame game minimizes the opportunities we have in life.

In his book *The Magic of Big Thinking*, David Schwartz lists four common forms of excusitis:

1. Health excusitis: "I don't feel good. I've got such-and-such wrong with me."

2. Intelligence excusitis: "I don't have the brains to succeed."

3. Age excusitis: "It's no use. I'm too old (or too young)."

4. Luck excusitis: "If it wasn't for bad luck, I'd have no luck at all!"

Schwartz says we all need to work to cure ourselves of excusitis because, like any disease, it gets worse if it isn't treated properly and keeps many of us stuck and stops us from fully enjoying our lives.

To help cure yourself of excusitis, consider the following **TIP**s:

• Refuse to talk about your health or worry about it.

- Be genuinely grateful for good health.

- Remember it is better to wear out than to rust out.

- Never underestimate your intelligence and never overestimate the intelligence of others.

- Remind yourself that your attitude is more important than your intelligence.

- Remember, the ability to think is of greater value than the ability to memorize facts.

- Know *stickability* is ninety-five percent of *ability*.

- Look at your present age positively.

- Accept and learn the laws of cause and effect.

- Never waste your mental muscles dreaming of an effortless way to win success.

Letting Go

No one is perfect. We all make mistakes and respond in ways that hurt others and ourselves. We hurt others through our actions, omissions and judgments and through our words, neglect and criticism. Letting go of the wrongs done to us and those we do to others improves our fun and our ability to play well.

> *"One of the secrets of a long and fruitful life is to forgive everybody, everything, every night before going to bed."*
>
> — Bernard M. Baruch (1870–1965), American financier and statesman

When we have been hurt by family or friends, some of us choose to hold a grudge and may even avoid interacting with them, becoming legalistic, rigid and merciless toward them. We hold onto the hurts we believe others have done to us and have great difficulty letting go of the past.

Seeking ways to understand or viewing situations from the other person's perspective can help us to let go of wrongs. Visualizing the person as a young child and understanding how they may have been hurt or mistreated assist us in seeing the situation and the person in a different light. In doing so, it becomes easier to be compassionate and let go of our negative feelings.

Not letting go can be likened to carrying a backpack full of rocks. Each unforgiven act increases the weight on our minds, making our journeys more difficult. It can be quite tiring to spend a lifetime carrying a heavy emotional load of hurtful acts by staying angry, resentful and bitter toward someone who in all probability does not know how we feel. By unloading these heavy thoughts, we let go of the offense and enable ourselves to live with greater ease, enjoyment and peace of mind.

When we experience hurt, harm or bitterness from someone's actions or words, negative feelings such as anger, confusion, sadness or even depression arise. Research has shown that not letting go can result in long-term health problems.[2]

In her book *Anatomy of the Spirit: The Seven Stages of Power and Healing*, Caroline Myss writes how the events in our lives, and how we respond to them, impact our physical health. She knows there is a strong link between physical and emotional stresses and specific illnesses—that certain emotional crises correspond specifically to certain parts of the body. She has observed that certain people who come to see her with a diagnosis of heart disease have had life experiences that block intimacy or love from their lives. She has seen how others with back pain have had persistent financial worries, and those with cancer have unresolved connections with the past, unfinished business and emotional issues. This observation has resulted in the idea that *cancer is the disease of unfinished business.*

---

2. Alex H.S. Harris and Carl E. Thoresen, "Forgiveness, Unforgiveness, Health, and Disease," in *Handbook of Forgiveness*, ed. Everett L. Worthington (New York: Routledge, 2005), 321–333, www.chce.research.va.gov/docs/pdfs/pi_publications/Harris/2005_Harris_Thorsen_HF.pdf.

In his book *Cancer Is Not a Disease, It's a Survival Mechanism*, Andreas Moritz, a medical intuitive from Germany, says cancer is one of the many ways the body forces us to change the way we see and treat ourselves and our bodies. He believes that constant conflicts, guilt and shame, which cause stress to our bodies, can easily paralyze our bodies' most basic functions and lead to the growth of a cancerous tumor.

Moritz has seen thousands of cancer patients over a period of three decades. In that time, he has come to recognize a certain pattern of thinking, believing and feeling common to most of his patients. He said he has "yet to meet a cancer patient who does not feel burdened by some poor self-image, unresolved conflict and worries, or past emotional conflict/trauma that still lingers in his subconscious mind and cellular memories." He believes the physical disease of cancer "cannot occur unless there is a strong undercurrent of emotional uneasiness and deep-seated frustration."

> "We blame little things in others and pass over great things in ourselves. We are quick enough in perceiving and weighing what we suffer from others, but we mind not what others suffer from us."
> — Thomas à Kempis (1380–1471), German Catholic monk and author

Effectively dealing with our emotions and letting go of our hurts can aid in alleviating emotional uneasiness and frustration.

Worry, Anxiety and Depression

The time we spend worrying is not fun time. When we worry, we spend time anticipating negative outcomes and lose touch with what is happening now. We are unable to see the good in the world and our surroundings. The world becomes a threatening place to us. However, most of our worries never come to pass.

Some of your hurts you have cured,
And the sharpest you still have survived,
But what torments of grief you endured
From evils which never arrived.

— Ralph Waldo Emerson (1803–1882),
American essayist, lecturer and poet

"Worry is a down payment on a problem you may never have."

— Joyce Meyer,
American charismatic,
author and speaker

Worry puts our focus on the future and alters our perceptions of life to the point where we lose our sense of reality. It twists neutral, everyday situations into nightmares.

Worry is a common temptation, and it is a favorite pastime for many. Some would even go so far as to imply that when we worry, we show we really care, but it actually shows we don't trust.

Worrisome thoughts can occupy a person's mind for a large part of the day, only to cause anxiety. Physically, worry and anxiety can feel like a tense knot in our stomachs or a pulling at our hearts. Mentally, it causes thoughts of dread to churn in our minds, tormenting us.

Webster's defines *worry* as "a mental distress or agitation resulting from concern usually for something impending or anticipated." Worry is tormenting oneself with disturbing thoughts—thoughts that may have no basis in reality. Worry won't lengthen our lives, but it may shorten them, and it will certainly snuff out our fun and effectiveness.

Charles Mayo, cofounder of the Mayo Clinic, observed how worry adversely affects our circulatory, endocrine and nervous systems. Mayo said he never knew anyone who died of overwork, but he knew many who died of worry. We can worry ourselves to death, but we will never worry ourselves into a longer life.

Have you ever heard someone say, "I'm worried sick"? Worrying can lead to sickness—stomach problems, ulcers, colon problems, headaches, nervous tension, stress, loss of sleep, loss of focus and forgetfulness.

Worry, left unresolved, will debilitate our minds and bodies. It becomes a thief, robbing us of our willingness to accept and enjoy life as it is. When we give into worry, we open a Pandora's box of terrifying pictures, sounds and events. We lose our foothold on reality as we attempt to control the terrible demons in our own anguished, private world.

Worry leads to anxiety. Anxiety disorders are a form of mental illness characterized by excessive, exaggerated anxiety and worry about everyday events with no obvious reasons. Anxious people expect disaster and cannot stop fretting about health, money, family, work or school. Anxiety over events and issues is often unrealistic or out of proportion to the situation, leading to a life lived in a constant state of fear and dread. Eventually, the worry and anxiety dominate our thinking to the point that it interferes with our day-to-day functioning. Our work, school and social endeavors, along with our relationships, are jeopardized.

When we are anxious, we are restless, irritable and have difficulty concentrating. We may experience muscle tension, headaches and sweating, along with nausea, increased urinary frequency and trouble sleeping. We may tire, tremble and be easily startled. Anxiety can lead to depression. Depression has been said to be "anger turned inward." It can lead to suicide, and that is definitely not fun for anyone.

According to the World Health Organization, suicide is one of the three leading causes of death among those aged fifteen to forty-four, and the second leading cause of death in those aged ten to twenty-four These figures do not include suicide attempts, which are up to twenty times more frequent than completed suicides.[3]

---

3. World Health Organization, "Mental Health: Suicide Prevention (SUPRE)," *SUPRE Publications* (2011), www.who.int/mental_health/prevention/suicide/ suicideprevent/en/.

Anxiety and depression are types of mental illness. The Canadian Mental Health Association (CMHA) cites studies that show one in every five Canadian adults under age sixty-five has a mental health problem.[4] Their studies do not include figures for those over age sixty-five.

Mental illness is not easy to understand. It is easier to comprehend and repair a broken limb than a broken mind, yet both are painful and debilitating. Mental illness is sometimes marked with fear and disgrace, resulting in hesitation to seek help and the potential for more destructive behaviors. It causes misery, tears and missed opportunities for the thousands affected by it.

Words like *crazy, cuckoo, psycho, wacko* and *nutso* keep the stigma of mental illness alive, belittling and offending individuals with mental health disorders. Following are some truths about mental illness:

- People with mental illness *are not* violent and dangerous: They are no more violent than any other person who is ill. In fact, they tend to be the victims of violence rather than to be violent themselves.

- People with mental illness *are not* poor or less intelligent: Studies have shown that most people dealing with mental illness are of average or above-average intelligence; mental illness, like physical illness, can affect anyone regardless of intelligence, social class or income.

- Mental illness *is not* caused by personal weakness: A diagnosis of mental illness is not a character flaw, nor is it about being weak or lacking willpower.

- Mental illness *is not* a single, rare disorder: Mental illness is a broad classification for many disorders. Anxiety, depression, eating disorders and organic brain disorders are forms of it. Mental illness also includes personality disorders such as

---

4. Canadian Mental Health Association (CMHA), "Understanding Mental Illness," CMHA Publication (2011), *www.cmha.ca/bins/content_page.asp?cid=3.*

schizophrenia, bipolar disorder, seasonal affective disorder (SAD), obsessive-compulsive disorder (OCD), phobias, panic attacks and post-traumatic stress disorder (PTSD).

CMHA uses the acronym **STOP** to educate others on ways to stop the fear and negative stigma behind mental illness and to aid in improved attitudes and actions to support those dealing with mental illness. It encourages everyone to **STOP**

- **S**tereotyping and assuming a standardized negative view of mental illness,

- **T**rivializing or belittling people with mental illness and/or the illness itself,

- **O**ffending and insulting those with mental illness, and

- **P**atronizing them by treating them as if they are not as good as other people.

"I Have a Secret!"

Sometimes worry, anxiety and depression are rooted in the secrets we keep—the skeletons in the family closet that we are never to mention, our mistakes in life that we fear will cause others to dislike us or social taboos or events we do not believe we can share with others. Secrets can be anything from our innermost thoughts and feelings to everyday events. Anything we believe we have to hide and cannot share with at least one other person has power over us. The energy we spend hiding our secrets takes away from the energy we could use to have fun.

Revealing our secrets to another person helps rid us of the burden of hiding them. It relieves the anxiety and stress of concealing and deceiving. It helps us to forgive ourselves and stop beating ourselves up. When we constantly remind ourselves of our secrets and past mistakes, it is like putting a ball and chain around our ankles, slowing our progress and dragging us down.

Gail Saltz, a psychiatrist at Weill Cornell Medical College and authority on the role secrets play in our lives, states, "Secrets are a fact of life. Everyone has them. But some secrets can carry a hidden price that affects both our psychological and physical health."

She goes on to say that keeping some thoughts and actions private helps us maintain the feeling that we are unique, but we may also keep secrets to avoid critical judgments by others and negative consequences. When we feel we cannot reveal some secrets, we begin to lead a secret life, and that becomes dangerous.

Sonya Visor, author of *Who I've Become Is Not Who I Am*, writes that "secrets cause inner conflict, creating anxiety, stress and worry." She says secrets affect us physically. They cause headaches, back pain, high blood pressure, digestive problems and depression. In extreme cases secrets lead to suicide.

A secret life develops when shame or guilt, along with the fear of consequences, creates a desperate need to keep aspects of our lives from becoming known. The problem with keeping others from discovering our secrets is that it requires constant vigilance. It leads to a life that revolves around various maneuvers to maintain a facade of normality. Hiding the fact that we did not give up smoking years ago and still have several cigarettes a day, that we lied on our résumés and never did go to college, that we have an addiction to Internet pornography or we cheated on our taxes requires a lot of energy.

Saltz says, "Self-exploration is the antidote to secrecy." She describes self-exploration as discovering our feelings and memories around our troubling behavior and understanding past events and relationships that may be controlling our behavior in the present.

Another key to successfully freeing ourselves from our secrets is to choose the right person to be our confidant. We need someone we can trust who can also bring new insight into our secrets. We need a person who will listen, be nonjudgmental and discreet, think constructively and help us get through the process of righting any wrongs the secrets may have caused.

We need to share our secrets, but not with someone who would be hurt by them. If your grandfather abused you forty years ago, and now your grandmother is eighty-five years old, it would not be wise to tell her what happened so many years ago. It may help you to release your secret, but it would burden her. It is best to find a trusted and wise friend or a well-trained therapist.

Sometimes we keep secrets from ourselves. Most of us are aware of *what* we are doing, but we are often unaware of *why* we are doing it. A man who has one affair after another can find ways to ensure no one knows about his activities. But is he aware of his own needs and the conflicts driving him to act in a way that could destroy his marriage?

What we refuse to know can also hurt our physical health in insidious ways. A woman who finds a breast lump and keeps forgetting to make an appointment with the doctor is hiding from herself the fear that it could be a sign of something serious. A man with high blood pressure who does not make the necessary diet and lifestyle changes has not faced the reality of his significantly higher risk of cardiovascular disease, a disease that may shorten his life.

Sharing our secrets with someone we trust has the same effect on our attitudes as daily hygiene has on our bodies. It gets rid of the poisons and impurities that invade our minds. When we hide parts of our lives, we build up toxic thoughts, which, over time, eat away at our health. Releasing them is a form of cleansing and washing away the guilt and shame.

Gossip

When someone has trusted you with their secret, how do you handle the information? Do you keep confidences and honor a person's right to privacy, or do you find someone to tell? Do you gossip? Gossip or criticism of others shows disrespect for them. Some of us may find gossip fun, but it does not add fun to the life of the person being gossiped about.

News used to be spread by word of mouth, letters and the printed word. Today the latest news about our friends and family has gone high tech with email, instant messaging and Facebook. We live in a culture where we can instantly voice our heated opinions in a public forum without the benefit of an editor or a permanent eraser.

In whatever way news is spread, if it is incorrect, unnecessary or hurtful, it is gossip. Gossip can tarnish a reputation even without a word being spoken. With a few keystrokes, someone's private information or a vicious rumor is on its way to hundreds, even thousands, of recipients.

Some of you may remember playing the telephone game when you were children. The game begins with one child whispering a message in the ear of the child sitting next to them. That child repeats the message in the ear of the next child, and so on until the information goes full circle, ending with the child who began it. The final player then reveals the message as they heard it and discloses what the original message had been. The discrepancy between the original and ending messages illustrates how information passed from one person to another becomes distorted. This is what happens when people gossip and share another's private information—wrong messages are passed on.

Gossip is everywhere, in the grocery store, the gym and the doctor's office. Gossip happens among groups of friends or peers, finds its way into the newspapers and sometimes it is considered national news. There are television shows and magazines that promote stories about others. Sharing someone's stories and secrets brings negative outcomes. It results in loss of trust, false assumptions, distorted facts and violated privacy, causing hurt feelings and damaged relationships.

You need **A B**etter **C**hoice to avoid gossip, such as the following:

- Stay focused on your life, your responsibilities and yourself. Use "I" statements when communicating with others, especially when communicating your thoughts and feelings.

- Agree not to hold conversations about someone who is not present.

- News bulletins, such as someone having a baby, going back to school or buying a new home, are allowed, but do not permit yourself to judge their decisions or speculate about their motives or the outcomes of their choices.
- Keep negative thoughts and knowledge about others to yourself.
- It takes two to gossip, so leave the room if you have to.
- Use the following examples of what to say in an uncomfortable gossip situation:
  - "I have to be honest. I don't think talking behind _____'s back about his/her problems is going to help him/her."
  - "As _____'s friends, I think we need to find better ways to support him/her instead of talking about him/her. Let's ask _____ how he/she would like us to support him/her."
  - "I'm uncomfortable discussing this. I know my feelings would be hurt if my friends were talking about my personal problems behind my back."

Addictive Behavior

When we hide our activities and behaviors from family and friends, we may think we do so to spare them worry, but we may actually do it because we have an addiction. Any activity, substance or behavior that has become the major focus of our lives, to the exclusion of other activities, or that has begun to harm us or others physically, mentally or socially, is considered to be an addiction.

Researchers have found similarities between physical addiction to various chemicals, such as alcohol and heroin, and psychological dependence on activities that become addictive behaviors, such as gambling, sex and shopping. These activities can also include working, exercising or eating or the use of technical devices such as cell phones and video games.

Addictive behaviors are rooted in our need to reduce the tension caused by our desire to avoid or control. Addictive behaviors are repetitive, seemingly purposeful and are often performed in a ritualistic manner. They are activities that are not connected to the purpose they are meant for, and they are likely to be excessive.

These activities produce endorphins in the brain, making us feel "high." Experts say that when we continue to engage in the activity to achieve a feeling of well-being and euphoria, we may get into an addictive cycle. In doing so, we become physically addicted to our own brain chemicals, leading to the continuation of the behavior, even though it may have negative health or social consequences.

Addictions lead to escalating deceit or secrets, cover-ups and detachment from ourselves. They result in harmful consequences that can be external, such as loss of a job, a car crash or divorce. The result could be internal, such as detachment, depression or lack of ability to feel or concentrate. There may also be physical consequences, such as illness, hypertension and memory loss.

Different addictive behaviors have a host of commonalities, making them more similar than different from each other and suggesting they need not be divided into separate diseases, categories or problems. Following are common tendencies associated with addictive behaviors. As you read them, ask yourself if you have any of these characteristics.

- Obsessing with and constantly thinking of the object, activity or substance

- Seeking out or engaging in the behavior, even though it is harmful

- Compulsively engaging in the activity—doing it over and over—even when you do not want to, and finding it difficult to stop

- Experiencing withdrawal symptoms such as irritability, cravings, restlessness and depression when you stop the activity

- Being unable to control when you engage in the behavior, or how long or how much

- Denying problems that result from your behaviors, even though others see the negative effects

- Hiding the behavior, even though family or close friends have mentioned their concern

- Reporting a blackout during the time you are engaged in the behavior

- Experiencing depression serious enough that you need to see a physician

- Experiencing low self-esteem and feeling anxious about not having control over your environment

- Coming from a psychologically or physically abusive families

Gratitude Changes Your Attitude

Being thankful for what we have and what we experience creates positive thinking, attitudes and energy and leads to more fun in our lives. Thankfulness builds us up and helps us see a better side of life. Thankfulness opens the door for good things to come into our lives. Saying thank you, making positive comments and engaging in affirmative conversations express our faith in our ability to improve life for the better or to make wiser choices.

Being thankful for what we already have received and accomplished, while pursuing

"Every reality you create in your life begins with what you imagine. So use the power of your imagination to imagine abundance, instead of focusing your thoughts on need. See yourself not as lacking, but as fulfilling. Let your thankfulness for what is possible crowd out any limiting thoughts."

— Ralph Marston, American author

what we want, opens windows of opportunity. Being thankful for the people in our lives, the ideas we have and the chance to work and produce results enhances life and health.

Financial experts and inspirational speakers agree that being grateful is a vital ingredient for increasing wealth and success in our lives. They say that by being grateful for the smaller and more immediate things, such as having a place to live, food to eat and air to breathe, we place ourselves in a positive frame of mind and open ourselves to pleasant and enjoyable aspects of healthful living.

When we are grateful, we attract good quality and higher standards. As we become more comfortable with the positive outcomes gratitude brings, we may even find ourselves feeling grateful for learning hard lessons and for our past mistakes. By being grateful, we lose our fears and begin to develop a deep appreciation for the wonderful and exciting adventure life really is. We will have more fun as our *gratitude changes our attitude*.

Be Thankful

Be thankful that you don't already have everything you desire.
If you did, what would there be to look forward to?
Be thankful when you don't know something,
For it gives you the opportunity to learn.
Be thankful for the difficult times.
During those times you grow.
Be thankful for your limitations,
Because they give you opportunities for improvement.
Be thankful for each new challenge,
Because it will build your strength and character.
Be thankful for your mistakes.
They will teach you valuable lessons.
Be thankful when you're tired and weary,

Because it means you've made the effort.
It's easy to be thankful for the good things.
A life of rich fulfillment comes to those who are
also thankful for the setbacks.
Gratitude can turn a negative into a positive.
Find a way to be thankful for your troubles,
and they can become your blessings.

— Author unknown

Embracing Health, Balance and Abundance through Fun

Taking the time to have fun, to play and to **L**augh **O**ut **L**oud lightens your life and reduces the impact of stress. It takes away the seriousness and tensions of life. A smile, a chuckle or a hearty laugh feels good and is good for your health. Having **FUN** brings friends into your life as well as **MAGIC**, as it **M**akes **A G**reat **I**mpact in **C**hanging your outlook.

Knowing what holds you back from having fun and fully enjoying your life is a way to increase the fun in your life. Your life is healthier and more stable when the fun you have is governed by your values and principles instead of excuses. To let go of your hurts and rid yourself of secrets and addictive behavior, you may find you need to **G**et **U**ncomfortable **T**o **S**ucceed, but in doing so, you improve your life. You will have more time and energy to engage in fun, play and laughter. It is all possible when you say ...

Let It Begin with Me!

Chapter 10

LIFE IS A DO-IT-YOURSELF PROJECT

You Are Responsible for You!

Remember, it is now believed that eighty percent of illness is stress related and that whatever our genetic weak link is, stress will trigger it.

Throughout this book, I have identified areas in life that may impact the stress, pressure and strain you encounter. As you strive to meet your daily needs, embracing health, balance and abundance with the support of your faith, family, fitness, friends, finance and fun will contribute to managing or decreasing your stress. The **TIP**s and **ABC**s offered will lend a hand in maintaining and improving your health and life. But how well this information

> *"Our very survival depends on our ability to stay awake, to adjust to new ideas, to remain vigilant and to face the challenge of change."*
> — Martin Luther King Jr. (1929–1968), American clergyman and activist

promotes your health depends on how well you take responsibility for yourself.

You are responsible for you. Your **R**eturn **O**n **L**ife will be proportionate to the quality of the investments you make in it. From a holistic perspective, it is the small daily choices, or investments, you make year after year that lead to the **ROL** you receive twenty, thirty or forty years down the road. If you don't make better choices throughout your life, it may be too late later on to reverse the impact and outcomes of your previous choices.

> *"If you want something you've never had, you must be willing to do something you've never done."*
>
> — Thomas Jefferson (1743–1826), principal author of the Declaration of Independence and third president of the United States

Our freedom of choice offers us the opportunity to improve ourselves, our health and our lives, or not. Day to day, these choices often seem too insignificant to influence outcomes. We make choices daily, unaware that they will alter us and the future of the generations that follow. The consequences are seldom fully understood at the time we make them. But they do come.

Consider the choices we make in the morning: We decide when to get up, what to eat and when to exercise. We decide on our mood and whether we will put a smile on our faces. Throughout the day, we make choices concerning what we will read, watch and listen to. We choose what we will say, comment on and avoid.

Every day, we may choose or not choose to learn something new and advance ourselves, to stay in our relationships or to be involved in our children's lives. We can choose our career paths and how to spend our days. We may choose to hope for better times, work for the greater good or see the positive in challenging situations.

The list of choices available to us each day is endless, and these small daily choices accumulate to impact our lives in significant ways.

Every choice we make is a choice not to do something else, even *a choice to do nothing is still a choice.*

By the time our days come to an end, we will have seen and accomplished much. We will have made choices that changed the direction of our lives and of other people's lives, some good and some not so good. We will have learned many lessons. We will have laughed and cried, worked toward our dreams, had family and friends

"The history of free men is never written by chance but by choice, their choice."
— Dwight D. Eisenhower (1890–1969), thirty-fourth president of the United States

come together and had family and friends pull away. We will have seen the passing of time and wondered why it went so slowly, and then in the next breath, wondered why it went so fast.

At our funerals, if we were able to speak to those we leave behind, what might we say? What choices would we encourage our family, friends and colleagues to make as they continue in their lives?

Each of us can make wiser choices to decrease our stress levels and experience a well-lived life, but that is an individual decision requiring knowledge and initiative. Remember, *if nothing changes, nothing changes.* I hope by reading this book you now have a greater awareness and respect for your choices and how the different areas of your life are impacted by them. Life is truly a do-it-yourself project. To live a rich, full life, you need to continually say, "Let it begin with me."

We have a responsibility to ourselves, our loved ones and society to **TAP** into our **T**alents, **A**bilities and **P**otential. It is up to each of us to know ourselves. It is our responsibility to change and grow, to become the best we can be and to be healthy in body, mind and soul.

Spiritual leader Emmet Fox said, "You are not happy because you are well. You are well because you are happy. You are not depressed because trouble has come to you, but trouble has come because you are depressed. You can change your thoughts and feelings, and then the outer things will change to correspond."

We need to be persistently aware of our thoughts and feelings. We need to examine and reflect on them as we learn to respond well to life, its challenges and its stresses so we stay healthy physically, mentally and spiritually. It doesn't take much to alter the course and outcome of our lives. We can change them for the better by developing an understanding of our strengths and weaknesses. Then we can create a personalized checklist of strategies to implement to balance our health and well-being as we keep our lives rolling smoothly.

> *"As human beings, our greatness lies not so much in being able to remake the world ... as in being able to remake ourselves."*
> — Mahatma Gandhi (1869–1948), Indian political and spiritual leader

Our lives can be beautiful and bountiful when we are willing to change, to prune ourselves and pull out the weeds that hinder us. We must plant, water and fertilize positive habits. We must consistently work at building and maintaining healthy relationships and practices. We can't sit back and rest on our laurels. Even when life is good, we must continue to work and be vigilant, as our imperfections may persistently resurface when our guard is down.

> *"Life is like riding a bicycle. To keep your balance you must keep moving."*
> — Albert Einstein (1879–1955), German theoretical physicist

It has been said that "our deepest fear is *not* that we are inadequate. Our deepest fear is that we are powerful beyond measure." We are "brilliant, gorgeous, talented and fabulous." We are magnificent masterpieces. We need to stop playing small and not allow ourselves to grow weak. We are all capable, gifted and full of great possibilities. But it takes **GUTS** to maintain balanced health and well-being. It takes courage and stamina to live well and bring out our true magnificence. It takes

- courage to become the best we can be;
- courage to step out of our comfort zones and take risks;
- stamina to maintain a healthy body, mind and soul;
- stamina for couples to continually work on maintaining a loving relationship in the face of adversity;
- courage for employees to improve themselves and learn new skills;
- courage for parents to teach their children how to live well and to say no to them;
- stamina for children to complete their studies, and courage to find their direction in life;
- courage for soldiers to go into battle to maintain our freedom;
- stamina to live a healthy and abundantly balanced life;
- courage to say, "Let it begin with me";
- courage to **TAP** into our **T**alents, **A**bilities and **P**otential, to learn, grow and change;
- courage to overcome the obstacles in life, to manage stress and say, "I can do this"; and
- courage and stamina to **G**et **U**ncomfortable **T**o **S**ucceed.

> *"No matter how you feel, get up, dress up and show up."*
>
> — Regina Brett, American columnist and author

"I Can Do This!"

Fear can stop us from reaching our potential. We may fear the uncertainty of change and the discomfort that often comes with change. But change is good. It keeps us fresh, growing and learning. Change prevents us from playing small. Don't be afraid to leverage the talent and potential you possess to further develop your abilities. *Don't ask for life to be made easier. Ask to be made better and stronger.*

We were created to enjoy diversity and variety. We have the ability to adapt and refresh our lives. Stepping out of our comfort zones and trying something new brings excitement and new experiences. We cannot change the seasons of our lives or many of the circumstances impacting our lives, but we can take personal responsibility to change ourselves and make the best of all our circumstances.

I have a friend whose family members are not permitted to say "I can't." They can say "I'll try" or "I tried and failed," but not "I can't." This family does not expect its members to be perfect, but they do expect each individual to make positive progress in their lives. They know that when someone else has accomplished a particular task or made a positive change in their life, it is possible for them to do so as well. They know that when they also work at something and learn how best to perform, they too can accomplish it.

> *"You can do anything in this world that you want to do, if you want it bad enough and you're willing to pay the price!"*
> — Mary Kay Ash (1918–2001), American businesswoman

To keep your health and life balanced and in shape, take actions to bring your desires to fruition. If you want better relationships, a different job or more finances, you can accomplish it. If you desire more travel or a fit body, you can achieve it when you are willing to put in the effort. You can do this! Don't hold yourself back. Become the best you can be in all areas of your life.

A friend said to me, "I reflected on a beautiful bouquet of flowers, inhaling the exquisite fragrance of the open blossoms and wishing the closed buds might open as well. But those buds didn't unfold to let go into their true magnificence."

She continued, "I realized that often I restrain myself from opening up into my true magnificence for fear that others will misunderstand and criticize me. But when I contemplated this idea in the context of flowers, I realized that holding back might mean hiding the beauty and creativity in me. This seemed like a sad misuse of my energy, just as each bloom in a bouquet of flowers is part of a whole that all together makes a beautiful symphony of color and fragrance."

She concluded, "It reminded me to relinquish my false reserve and allow my own particular blooms to develop to their brightest and most fragrant so that I could claim my rightful place in the bouquet of people around me."

Let your life blossom. Make **A B**etter **C**hoice and learn **TIP**s **T**o **I**mprove your **P**erformance in life by asking yourself these questions:

- What am I doing with what I've got?
- What can I accomplish?
- What can I learn?
- What can I read?
- Whom can I ask?
- What more do I want from life?

> *"Everyone thinks of changing the world, but no one thinks of changing himself."*
> — Leo Tolstoy (1828–1910), Russian author

Why are we so reluctant to make different choices for our lives and change? Why do we have a tendency to wait for things to happen instead of being proactive and initiating the change that we want? The answer may be found in the **Three P's**: **P**erfection, **P**rocrastination and **P**aralysis. When we wait for the **P**erfect time, place and situation, or **P**rocrastinate by making excuses for our inability to forge ahead, we may become **P**aralyzed and never adapt enough to achieve our goals.

In reality, we are not required to be **P**erfect in what we do. Change and moving forward calls us to take that first awkward step and then continue to make progress. It's about trying and doing, not being **P**erfect. *When we* **P**rocrastinate, *we don't avoid the pain, we just defer it.* We do not need to remain **P**aralyzed by freezing and doing nothing. Changing our attitudes and saying, "Let it begin with me" works best. Then, just do it!

Perfectionism and procrastination stop us from engaging in activities and practices that bring us better lives and health. They stop us from saying yes to new opportunities. Remember, *there never was a winner who wasn't first a beginner.*

To overcome the **Three P's**, the **Three C's** reinforce the reality that change is rarely an event, but a process—a process that begins with Confusion, leading us to Comfort and, inevitably, to new Capabilities.

When we start anew, there will be a short time of self-doubt and apprehension. But when we persevere, this Confusion doesn't last and we adapt and become more Comfortable with the new situation. Before we know it, in a relatively short time, we are Capable. With each new step, we changed, grew and improved.

> **"Man is made or unmade by himself."**
>
> — James Allen (1864–1912), British author and pioneer of the self-help movement

Those who understand the process of the **Three C's** risk more, do more and learn more. Confusion is a small price to pay for the return we ultimately receive. Laugh with others, or by yourself, at the challenges of new beginnings, knowing you're not alone in experiencing them. In doing so, you will feel more Comfortable in continuing and persevering until you are truly Capable. An I-can-do-this attitude will propel you into a world of new possibilities.

> **"The future is not some place we are going to, but one we are creating."**
>
> — John Schaar (1928–2011), American scholar and political theorist

Chris Widener, a well-known motivational speaker, says, "Life does not reward thinking. Life rewards action. Let me clarify: Life rewards thoughtful action. Think first, by all means, but then ACT! Anything you want to accomplish will only be done by bold and decisive action." In other words, just do it!

Remember, because of **FEAR**, we may **F**orget **E**verything **A**nd **R**un. But also remember, **FEAR** is **F**alse **E**vidence **A**ppearing **R**eal. While seeking to make everyday decisions, many of us focus on our fears and what may go wrong by saying, "What if I mess up?" "What if I can't do this?" "What if I am wrong?" By focusing on what may go wrong, we get caught up in our inabilities and past errors, paralyzing our efforts and losing sight of our capabilities and potential.

Fear of responsibility, being judged and what people will think can stop us. Fear of failure and criticism, along with fear of sacrifice or hard work, will stop us from doing what we need or want to do. Put **FEAR** to rest by

- **F**ocusing on what you have previously accomplished,

- **E**xploring all the possibilities,

- **A**sking for assistance, and

- **R**esolving to be persistent and positive as you trust the process.

> *"We must believe that we are gifted for something, and that this thing, at whatever cost, must be attained."*
>
> — Marie Curie (1867–1934), French-Polish physicist, chemist and two-time Nobel Prize recipient

The Buddy System

Being accountable to someone can help alleviate our fears and keep us on track as we progress in the direction we set for ourselves. The primary purpose of accountability is to encourage and strengthen ourselves, but it involves confronting our flaws.

Some of us may not value the importance of accountability because we put greater value on our independence and freedom. We put limits on the significance of our commitments and responsibilities to ourselves, others and society. We don't enjoy being questioned by others on what we do and how we live.

Accountability is actually a form of protection. It keeps us honest, focused and, ultimately, guards us from painful consequences. Laws exist for our protection and the protection of others. When we do not follow these laws, we hurt ourselves and others. Similarly, there are guidelines, or best practices for living life, that are embodied in good health practices, spiritual doctrines, psychiatry books, self-help manuals and our own hearts, but they are not enforceable. Being *obedient to the unenforceable* and doing the *must* do, not the *wanna* do, are important yet unenforceable laws.

Just as we are accountable to follow the laws of our society and for our performance at work, being accountable to others for how we perform helps us manage our fears and assists us to evolve into the person we are meant to be.

> *"Denying or refusing to deal with some unpleasant fact in your life is the source of most stress and unhappiness."*
>
> — Brian Tracy, Canadian author and motivational speaker

Accountability begins at home. Husbands and wives are accountable to each other. Children are accountable to their parents, teachers and other authority figures who guide them to become responsible adults. Friends are accountable to friends.

Politicians are accountable to citizens. Employees are accountable to employers. Would you want to drive over a bridge built by workers who answered to no one? We need the safeguard of trustworthy individuals who show up on time, put in an honest day's work and do their best, even when no one is watching.

Governments are founded on the idea that we can't simply do as we please. We need order. Laws must be obeyed and taxes must be paid to strengthen our country and not tear it down. The same is true for us. We will be better people when we embrace accountability for the lives we choose to live.

When you reach the end of your life, will you feel good about how you lived your life? Will you look back at your achievements and your impact on the world with a sense of pride and accomplishment, saying, "Well done," or will you look back with regrets because you were afraid or made unwise choices? Being accountable to others facilitates a better **ROL**, a better **Return On your Life**.

It is easier to remain accountable daily and correct our actions before they go out of control. You can improve your accountability performance by

- reviewing your day before going to sleep every night—looking at what you did and what you neglected to do, and then asking yourself what requires correction or improvement;

- making a decision to meet a wise and trusted mentor weekly or monthly to discuss the various aspects of your life and discover ways to enhance them;

- considering accountability to a higher spirit as you follow set guidelines that embody your values and principles; and

- remaining mindful of the children's verse "Good, better, best, never let it rest 'til your good is better and your better is best!"

"I Have a Dream!"

Having a dream and a purpose to pursue changes us; it empowers us and helps us grow. Think how the dreams of the following people empowered them:

- Walt Disney: To make people happy

- Henry Ford: To mass produce, mass distribute and mass sell cars

- Andrew Carnegie: To manufacture and market steel

- Mother Teresa: To care for and comfort the poor, sick and needy

> *"When a dream takes hold of you, what can you do? You can run with it, let it run your life, or let it go and think for the rest of your life about what might have been."*
>
> — Patch Adams, American physician and speaker

Dreams don't need to be big, but having one gives us a new perspective on life. Dreams motivate us to learn and experience new things, meet new people and consider new ways. Dreams are the fuel to push our lives in new directions as we make different choices and change.

Dreams infuse a positive focus into our lives. When we pursue a dream, we no longer dwell on disturbing matters or seek to solve issues beyond our control. Dreams give us an opportunity to pull away and focus on something other than our problems. They refresh our thoughts and uplift us as we see life in a new light. A creative project, a new interest or pursing new possibilities is like healing medicine.

With purpose and a dream, we see the world around us and ask, "What can I do with my time, abilities and energy to reach my potential?" "What can I do to make a difference, to have an impact?"

> *"If one advances confidently in the direction of his dreams, and endeavors to live the life which he has imagined, he will meet with a success unexpected in common hours."*
>
> — Henry David Thoreau (1817–1862), American author, poet and philosopher

Graveyards can be sad places. They are filled with books never written, songs never sung and words never spoken. Graveyards are full of projects never completed and dreams never met. Many people die without having pursued their dreams. They did not live to see what they were capable of accomplishing.

When we fail to pursue our dreams, live up to our potential or discover what we can do, a part of us dies. We separate ourselves from opportunities and living to our fullest potential. We stop striving to be the best we can be, the person we were meant to be. Don't rob the world of your amazing gifts by taking them to the grave with you. *Don't die with your music still inside you.*

Living life with purpose has been shown to cut our risk of Alzheimer's disease in half. Dr. Patricia Boyle, a researcher at Rush University Medical Center in Chicago, tracked more than 900 older persons without Alzheimer's disease for four years. Each person was asked periodically to rate themselves on a scale of 1 to 10 with questions such as "Do I enjoy making plans for the future and working toward making them real?" or "Do I feel good when I think of what I've done in the past and what I hope to do in the future?" By the end of the study, more than 155 of 951 participants developed Alzheimer's. This group was correlated to those who had a lower purpose in their lives. The participants who set concrete goals, maintained plans and lived with a purpose experienced better health.

Dr. Boyle found that patients with purpose and dreams were thirty percent less likely to have a heart attack. They also had lower cholesterol levels, fewer chronic medical conditions and showed fewer symptoms of depression. They had lower waist-to-hip ratios; in other words, people who led a high-purpose life were slimmer. The study confirmed that being purpose-driven helps protect us from health problems.[1]

Surveys tell us that nearly half of all adults admit they are seeking to understand the meaning and ultimate purpose of their lives. Researchers have confirmed that more than three out of every four adults want to make a difference in the world and want lives that count for some lasting, positive outcome. But most people hold onto their desires as something to experience in the future; it's not a present reality for them. Many do not take time to know the cause, purpose or dream that will give their life genuine fulfillment.

> *"Whatever you can do or dream you can, begin it. Boldness has genius, power and magic in it."*
>
> — Johann Wolfgang von Goethe (1749-1832), German writer, artist and politician

The key is to begin—to stop waiting for the perfect time and circumstances, to stop procrastinating and stop being paralyzed.

---

1. Patricia A. Boyle, Aron S. Buchman, Lisa L. Barnes, and David A. Bennett, "Effect of a Purpose in Life on Risk of Incident Alzheimer Disease and Mild Cognitive Impairment in Community-Dwelling Older Persons," *Archives of General Psychiatry* 67, no. 3 (2010): 304–310.

> *"A great deal of talent is lost in the world for want of a little courage ... The fact is that to do anything in the world worth doing, we must not stand back shivering and thinking of the cold and danger, but jump in and scramble through as well as we can."*
>
> — Sydney Smith (1771–1845), English clergyman, critic, philosopher and wit

> *"Our lives begin to end the day we become silent about things that matter."*
>
> — Martin Luther King Jr. (1929–1968), American clergyman and activist

Committing to a purpose leads to a new level of satisfaction and significance in your life. If you don't have a purpose, you could say your first purpose is to find a purpose or a **DREAM** that motivates you to

- **D**are to pursue your purpose,
- **R**elentlessly strive for
- **E**xcellence and
- **A**bandon alternate plans, while consistently
- **M**easuring how you are bringing your purpose, goals and dreams to fruition.

When you don't know where to begin, serving and helping others is a great place to start. In so doing, you may find you are the one who has been helped and a dream has developed. One of my friends began serving on a committee at the hospital where she worked. She enjoyed being involved and meeting new people. As time passed, she was asked to take part in another project—one act of service had led to another. This project was to implement a program called Prevent Alcohol and Risk-related Trauma in Youth (PARTY), which helped young people get through their teen years and beyond by showing them how to make smart choices.

In order to facilitate this program, my friend attended information sessions. While attending the first session, she met people who, unfortunately, had made some bad choices. She met others who, unfortunately, had someone else make a bad choice for them and were now living with the consequences. Meeting these people and hearing their stories stirred something inside her. My friend became excited and passionate as she realized the PARTY program was giving her a purpose and a dream to continue serving and helping.

Say Yes!

Another friend and I met for coffee. She told me that for years she had dreamed of taking a five-week vacation to walk *el Camino de Santiago*, a pilgrimage route through northwest Spain. She had saved the money to take the vacation, but she had yet to go. Even though she was entitled to only three weeks' paid vacation, her place of employment would grant her the full five weeks needed to walk the route. She would lose two weeks' pay. Money—taking two weeks off work without pay—was her biggest obstacle.

> *"Twenty years from now you will be more disappointed by the things you didn't do than by the ones you did do."*
>
> — Mark Twain (1835–1910), American author and humorist

As we spoke about the trip and how special it would be for her to go, a big smile shone on her face, a glow came to her cheeks and a twinkle gleamed in her eyes. We discussed ways she could overcome her obstacle of two weeks' unpaid leave. With some minor adjustments to her budget and to her thinking, she could take her dream vacation. We began to laugh as she made the choice to walk el Camino—to say yes!

When we stop playing small, living begins to happen. When we change our thoughts, views and actions, life explodes with possibility.

Making these changes by releasing old thoughts, habits and actions is difficult, but truly living life is impossible when you never begin. Begin **NOW** and let **N**o **O**pportunity be **W**asted. Start something **NEW** so **N**o **E**xperience is **W**asted. Improve **LIFE** as you begin to **L**ive **I**ntentionally **F**or **E**xcellence.

You may ask, "But **HOW** am I to begin? Where do I start?" The answer is that changing old behaviors and habits begins when you are

- **H**onest with yourself,
- **O**pen to new ways and ideas, and
- **W**illing to try new approaches and behaviors.

> *"As long as you live, keep learning how to live!"*
>
> — Seneca (4 BCE–CE 65), Roman philosopher, statesman and dramatist

When we change **HOW** we think, **HOW** we prioritize and **HOW** we react to life's opportunities and challenges, we begin to **L**ive **I**ntentionally **F**or **E**xcellence. My friend became **H**onest with herself and her desire to experience this special trip. She became **O**pen to new ways to manage her finances and her attitude and became **W**illing to assume the risk of an unpaid leave in order fulfill a dream. She began to say yes!

> *"Say yes / Life keeps happenin' every day / Say yes / When opportunity comes your way / You can't start wonderin' what to say / You'll never win if you never play / Say yes."*
>
> — Fred Ebb and John Kander, American musical theater lyricists

In his book *The Slight Edge*, Jeff Olson wrote, "It only takes five years to turn your life completely around. But it will take you the rest of your life to continue living like you are." I read this line in 1997 when my life was in turmoil. I did not like myself or my life. I was recovering from my first diagnosed episode of mental illness, my second marriage was breaking down and my finances were a mess. I had been on sick leave for ten months, and my benefits were running out. I lived far away from family and friends and found myself in a women's shelter with three children ages four, eleven and fifteen. I was forty-three years old and thought, "How did I get myself into this predicament?" "How did my life become such a mess?"

Jeff's quote gave me hope. It opened me to the fact that I could take charge of the realities of my life. I created a dream where I would change my ways, my thoughts and my life to improve it for my children and myself. I said yes to the **H**onesty, **O**penness and **W**illingness necessary to change my choices and improve my five-year **ROL**. I learned new ways and persevered; I began by saying yes to change.

By 2002 my life was different, and it was better. So I said yes to another five years, and then again to another five. My life has changed immensely since I first read the advice of Jeff Olson. I did the work to confront difficulties by being honest with myself and open to new approaches. With willingness, I set out to develop a healthier and better me.

November 2012 completed fifteen years since I committed to change. It has been an intriguing journey, with many unexpected twists and turns. I made the choice to live my dreams. I refused to experience life as a death sentence, separated from living.

But life was rarely easy. With each new experience, I strove to overcome my fears and focus on the positive. There was always a lesson to learn, a new wisdom or an aha moment to enhance life. There were many times I was afraid, nervous or anxious. I often felt insecure about what I was doing or needed to do, but I persevered and did not quit. Now, I continue to advance forward, as neither I nor any situation calls for perfection. I just say yes!

> *"We are here to laugh at the odds and live our lives so well that Death will tremble to take us."*
>
> — Charles Bukowski (1920–1994), American poet and novelist

Persistence

It is easier to begin something than to finish it. When we begin something new, we are excited and receive enthusiastic support from others. But as the days go by and our purpose becomes a daily matter of consistent hard work, and sometimes drudgery, enthusiasm subsides.

We are often left with nobody to urge us on except ourselves. Troubles and challenges come to discourage, frustrate and overwhelm us. We must consistently decide to see it through to the finish. We must persevere.

> "Continuous effort—
> not strength or
> intelligence—is the
> key to unlocking our
> potential."
> — Winston Churchill
> (1874–1965), British
> politician and statesman

If we were to choose just one personality trait to develop that would guarantee our success, placing persistence at the top of our lists would be our best choice. In his book *Think and Grow Rich*, Napoleon Hill stated, "There may be no heroic connotation to the word *persistence*, but the quality is to the character of man, what carbon is to steel." As Hill studied the world's most successful people, he found the quality they all shared was persistence. They would not give up. When successful people fail, they see it as a temporary inconvenience, a learning experience, an isolated event and a stepping-stone instead of a stumbling block.

Many athletes become successful because they don't give up. People who overcome obstacles succeed because they persist. They know obstacles can slow us down, but they ask us to triumph over them.

> "We are what we
> repeatedly do.
> Excellence, then, is
> not an act, but
> a habit."
> — Aristotle (384–322
> BCE), Greek philosopher

Developing persistence requires desire. Desire arouses enthusiasm for what we want to accomplish. *The depth of our desire impacts the swiftness of our progress.* When our desire is weak, our achievements will be few. When our desire is strong and we are persistent and willing to do what it takes, our achievements will be many.

When it comes to living a healthy and abundantly balanced life, what is your depth of desire to achieve it? What types of investments are you willing to make in your life in order to succeed? What is your depth of desire to build and maintain your health, reduce stress and prevent disease?

What is your depth of desire to develop a healthy **F**aith in yourself, in others, in life processes and in a higher spirit? Are you willing to move out of your comfort zone, develop your special talents and create a purpose for your life? Are you willing to overcome obstacles?

What is your depth of desire to build better relationships with your **F**amily members? Are you willing to spend time with them, talk to them and support them? Are you willing to accept your family members for who they are and to forgive their indiscretions?

What is your depth of desire to improve and maintain a healthy **F**itness level for your body, mind and soul? Are you willing to exercise regularly and consume healthful food and drink? Are you willing to maintain a clean environment? Are you willing to embrace a positive attitude as you manage your thoughts and emotions?

What is your depth of desire to put in the time and energy to acquire **F**riends who are supportive, dependable and healthy for you? Are you willing to become involved with others? Are you willing to be your own best friend?

What is your depth of desire to build long-term security by managing your **F**inances well? Are you willing to use a budget and say no to items you do not need? Are you willing to seek the aid of good financial counsel? Are you willing to encourage and teach your children to be self-supporting?

What is your depth of desire to create healthful **F**un in your life? Are you willing to develop a positive and grateful attitude? Are you willing to stand behind your principles and values and **TAP** into your **T**alents, **A**bilities and **P**otential?

Do you have the depth of desire to persist in achieving a life well lived? Are you willing to take an honest look at yourself

> *"The reality is, success rarely 'shows up'; it is lured and attracted day by day, by the right actions, thinking, and heart."*
>
> — Doug Firebaugh, American trainer, speaker and author

and your life and say, "Let it begin with me"? Are you willing to stay focused and not make excuses? You cannot receive the *perks* in life without doing the *works*. To experience all the wonders life has to offer, are you willing to do the work?

As you review your level of health and well-being and your balance and abundance within each of the **Six F's**, ask yourself, "Is the way I am living working for me?" To succeed, you need to persist. You need to maintain your desire. When you give up, you cheat yourself and others out of what could have been. Commit to persevering. At times you will feel as though you're spinning your wheels and will question whether you made the right choice or if you are on the right track. But remember, you will always get out of the ruts and make your way through the potholes of life when you stay committed, trust the process and persevere.

Find guidance in making the right decision and ask for the fortitude to cling to your decisions against all pressures and persuasions. Stop, rest and refresh yourself, but pick up where you left off and keep moving. You will experience ups and downs and may even feel like a **YOYO**. Know that to fully accomplish the desires for your life, **You're On Your Own**. Your life is a do-it-yourself project. Persevere and do not quit.

When things go wrong, as they sometimes will,
When the road you're trudging seems all uphill,
When the funds are low and the debts are high,
And you want to smile, but you have to sigh,
When care is pressing you down a bit,
Rest, if you must, but don't you quit.

Life is queer with its twists and turns,
As every one of us sometimes learns,
And many a failure turns about,

When he might have won had he stuck it out;
Don't give up though the pace seems slow—
You may succeed with another blow.

Often the goal is nearer than
It seems to a faint and faltering man,
Often the struggler has given up,
When he might have captured the victor's cup,
And he learned too late when the night slipped down,
How close he was to the golden crown.

Success is failure turned inside out—
The silver tint of the clouds of doubt,
And you never can tell how close you are,
It may be near when it seems so far,
So stick to the fight when you're hardest hit—
It's when things seem worst that you must not quit.

— **Author unknown**

Remind yourself to focus on the bigger picture; focus on the end results and think about the outcomes if you were to quit. Know that when you quit and stop persevering, you will not succeed. When you quit, you will always wonder if you could have succeeded. You will always ask, "What if I had succeeded in fulfilling my dreams?" Do not quit. Persevere and just do it!

Let It Begin with Me!

A doctor gave his patients a prescription. It read: "Repeat three times every morning, noon and night for the rest of your life: 'Every day, in every way, I am getting better and better!'" His patients received such marvelous results that people traveled from all over the world to avail themselves of this doctor's services.

Living a healthy and abundantly balanced life begins with you. It is up to you, no one can reach your potential for you. No one else can maintain or improve your health or overcome your challenges and obstacles, reduce your stress or prevent your disease. It starts with you.

Consider how your biography, your life story, affects your life and health. When you strengthen your relationships with **F**amily and **F**riends, build a stronger **F**aith, enhance your **F**itness and your **F**inances or simply have more **F**un, your life will be better. When you make wiser choices, eliminate excuses and develop a positive attitude, you enrich your health and life and help avert disease.

Life is challenging, but we grow strong and resilient through trials. The lessons teach us what works for our good and the good of others. They teach us to be wiser, build our characters and mold ourselves into better human beings. When life becomes difficult, don't deaden yourself. Don't look for the easy way out. Don't play small.

The popular music group Bon Jovi sings, "It's my life / It's **NOW** or never / I ain't gonna live forever." Say yes to life. Say yes to change. Say yes to the opportunities and experiences that come your way. Begin at some point on your balance wheel of health and well-being. Choose one of the **Six F's** where there is stress, or one you feel drawn to, or simply pick a spot at random. Just begin.

Challenge yourself to persistently uphold and upgrade your life in order to live it to the fullest. When you begin to falter, take time to reflect on the shape of your balance wheel, search for ways to bring yourself back to a steady momentum. Use the acronyms or a **TIP**, find **A B**etter **C**hoice or read an inspirational verse as you find a sound health and life practice that works for you. Make the needed adjustments. Don't let a misspent biography become an unhealthy and diseased biology.

There is another "I" statement exercise in appendix IV and another balance wheel of health and well-being exercise in appendix V. I encourage you to redo these exercises after you complete this book. Perhaps while reading **GUTS** your life changed. Perhaps you feel more balanced. Perhaps your attitude is different. Redo the exercises again in several months, in a year and every few years for the rest of your life. Consider using some of the strategies outlined in this book, or find other proven life and health strategies. Use them to plan a better **LIFE** for yourself and your loved ones as you continually **L**ive **I**ntentionally **F**or **E**xcellence.

> *"What is the use of living if it be not to strive for noble causes and to make this world a better place for those who will live in it after we are gone?"*
> — Winston Churchill (1874–1965), British politician and statesman

I challenge you to rise each morning with a positive attitude and do your best. Persevere as you cultivate your **F**aith, **F**amily, **F**itness, **F**riends, **F**inance and **F**un in ways that minimize stress and enhance living. Say thank you. Don't let your inabilities, imperfections or past become your focus; build on your potential. You do not need to know all the answers, what the future holds or the entire path you will follow. Just begin and stay positive and open-minded. Enjoy the experience and you will do well. Pursue your dreams and love the magnificent masterpiece you and those around you are. Remember,

People are unreasonable, illogical and self-centered,
Love them anyway.
If you do good, people will accuse you of selfish, ulterior motives,
Do good anyway.
If you are successful, you win false friends and true enemies,
Succeed anyway.
Honesty and frankness make you vulnerable,
Be honest and frank anyway.
What you spent years building may be destroyed overnight,
Build anyway.
People really need help but may attack you if you help them,

Help people anyway.
Give the world the best you have and you'll get kicked for it,
Give the world the best you have anyway.
The good you do today may be forgotten tomorrow,
Do good anyway.
Give the world the best you have, and it may never be enough,
Give your best anyway.
For in the end, it is between you and God.
It never was between you and them anyway.

— **Mother Teresa (1910–1997),**
Albanian Roman Catholic nun, founder
of the Missionaries of Charity

When it is time to lay you to rest, I hope many will come to rejoice and celebrate the abundance of your life. I pray you will have accomplished great successes. When you reach the end of your life, I trust you will be content with the life you lived, that you lived it well, free of regrets. I hope you will be at peace and all who know and love you will share that peace.

As you live, continue to say, "Let it begin with me." Let it be a constant reminder to seek new and better ways. You are responsible for you! Make your life a do-it-yourself project. Embrace the process of change. Search out what you are capable of accomplishing; know your potential and then begin to reach for it. Don't be afraid, don't hold back, say yes and, please, do not quit. Demonstrate your intestinal fortitude and **G**et **U**ncomfortable **T**o **S**ucceed.

Become the best you can be within each of the Six F's. Embrace and live a healthy life that is abundantly balanced as you continually say ...

Let It Begin with **ME**!

Appendix I

ACRONYMS

A's, the Three: Awareness, Acceptance, Action

ABC: A Better Choice
Always Be Courteous

ANTS: Angry Negative ThoughtS

BAG: Blessings, Accomplishments, Goals

BEST: Bless, Edify, Share, Touch
Bless, Encourage, Share, Time

BFF: Best Friend Forever

BIBLE: Basic Instruction Before Leaving Earth

CAT: Communication, Autonomy, Trust

C's, the Three: Confusion, Comfort, Capabilities

COMMUNICATE: Care, Openness, Mean what you say, Mutual respect, Understand, Nurture, Individuality, Clarify, Actively listen, Trust, Encourage

CORE: Compassion, Orderly behavior, Respect, Empathy

DEATH: Delivering Earth's Angels To Heaven

DENIAL: Don't Even Notice I Am Lying

DETACH: Don't Ever Think About Changing Him/Her

DINS:	Dual Income, No Sex
DREAM:	Dare to pursue a purpose, Relentlessly strive for Excellence and Abandon alternate plans, while consistently Measuring how you are bringing your purpose, goals and dreams to fruition
EGO:	Ease God Out
F's, the Six:	Faith, Family, Fitness, Friends, Finance, Fun
FAMILY:	Father And Mother, I Love You
FEAR:	False Evidence Appearing Real
	Forget Everything And Run
	Focus, Explore, Ask, Resolve
FINE:	F'd up, Insecure, Neurotic, Emotional
FORM:	Family, Occupation, Recreation, Message
GOALS:	God's Objectives Always Lead to Success
GOD:	Good Orderly Direction
GUTS:	Get Uncomfortable To Succeed
HALT:	Hungry, Angry, Lonely, Tired
HOPE:	Help Other People Excel
	Help Others Pursue Excellence
	Help Other People Escape
	Help Others Pursue Education
HOW:	Honest, Open, Willing
in-to-me-see:	intimacy
IOU:	I Over You
JOB:	Just Over Broke
KASH:	Knowledge, Attitude, Skills, Habits
KISS:	Keep It Super Simple
LIAR:	Let's Inspire Another Response
LIES:	Limiting Ideas that Eliminate Success

LIFE: Live Intentionally For Excellence

LOL: Lots Of Love

Laugh Out Loud

LOVE: Listen, Overlook, Validate, Effort

Learn, Overlook, Value, Energy

LUCK: Labor Under Correct Knowledge

MAD: Modern American Diet

MAGIC: Make A Great Impacting Change

MYOB: Mind Your Own Business

NEW: No Experience Wasted

NFL: No Friends Left

NOW: No Opportunity Wasted

P's, the Three: Perfection, Procrastination, Paralysis

PMS: Poverty Mentality Syndrome

PUSH: Pray Until Something Happens

REST: Remember, Entrust, Stand firm, Take the lessons

ROI: Return On Investment

ROL: Return On Life

SERVICE: Self-esteem, Experience, Respect, Validation, Ideas, Confidence, Excellence

SMART: Specific, Measurable, Attainable, Realistic, Timely

STOP: Stereotyping, Trivializing, Offending, Patronizing

TAP: Talent, Ability, Potential

TEAM: Together Everyone Achieves More

Together Excellence, Alone Mediocrity

THINK: Thoughtful, Honest, Intelligent, Necessary, Kind

TIP: To Improve Performance

WIN: What's Important Now?

YOYO: You're On Your Own

PEARLS OF WISDOM

1. Your biography becomes your biology. — Carolyn Myss

2. He who knows others is learned; he who knows himself is wise. — Lao-Tzu

3. As long as you live, keep learning how to live. — Seneca

4. Know thyself. — Socrates

5. An ounce of prevention is worth a pound of cure.

6. If you do what you've always done, you'll get what you always got. — Mark Twain

7. The source of our personal power is our beliefs.

8. The only thing that separates any one of us from excellence is fear, and the opposite of fear is faith. — Michael J. Fox

9. Feel the fear and do it anyway.

10. Fear knocked on my door. When faith answered, no one was there.

11. Don't fear to go out on a limb, that is where the fruit is. — H. Jackson Brown Jr.

12. There never was a winner who wasn't first a beginner.

13. By the inch, success is a cinch; by the yard, it's hard.

14. A man who carries a cat by the tail learns something he can learn in no other way. — Mark Twain

15. Instead of minding other people's business, create some business of your own to mind.

16. Practice makes perfect.

17. Whoever is out of patience is out of possession of his soul. — Jonathan Swift

18. Life does not happen in our time; it happens in due time.

19. Don't throw out the baby with the bath water.

20. Seeking God's presence and not God's presents leads to peace of mind.

21. Prayer is faith in action.

22. Love is to let those we love be perfectly themselves, and not to twist them to fit our own image. — Thomas Merton.

23. Love is not a feeling; it is an act of the will.

24. Family is a "we" thing, not a "me" thing.

25. It's not about finding the right person; it's also about being the right person.

26. No one wins unless you both do.

27. I'll take care of me for you and you take care of you for me.

28. The best inheritance you can leave your children is to be a good example. — Barry Spilchuk

29. It is easier to build strong children than to repair broken men. — Frederick Douglass

30. Consider how the letters in the word *listen* are the same as those in *silent*.

31. No is a complete sentence not requiring a defence or justification.

32. To truly love the adult you are, you need to own the child you were.

33. Alcoholism is a family disease.

34. When we hold onto hurt, we hand control of our emotions to another person.

35. Hurt people hurt people.

36. Bend and stretch, reach for the sky, stand on tippy toes, oh so high!

37. A man's health can be judged by which he takes two of at a time—pills or stairs. — Joan Welsh

38. Smile and the whole world smiles with you.

39. You are what you eat. — Victor Hugo Lindlahr

40. You create your entire life with your thoughts. — Brian Tracy.

41. Always free, always safe, always secure.

42. To compare is to despair.

43. Serenity Prayer: God, grant me the serenity to accept the things I cannot change, the courage to change the things I can, and the wisdom to know the difference. — Reinhold Niebuhr

44. It is a wealthy person indeed who calculates riches not in gold, but in friends. — Jim Stovall

45. Be careful of the friends you choose, for you will become like them. — W. Clement Stone

46. Surround yourself with people most like the person you want to become. — Tom Hopkins

47. To have a friend, be a friend.

48. People are lonely because they build walls instead of bridges. — Joseph F. Newton

49. Point one finger at another, then check to see how many fingers are pointing back at you.

50. *Anger* is one letter short of *danger*.

51. There is no winning an argument, but everyone wins an agreement.

52. Seek first to understand.

53. The only ones among you who will be happy are those who will have sought and found how to serve. — Albert Schweitzer

54. As we give to others, our giving gives back.

55. The only way to be truly satisfied is to do what you believe is great work; the only way to do great work is to love what you do. — Steve Jobs

56. Life is ten percent how you make it and ninety percent how you take it.

57. The highest reward for a person's toil is not what they get for it, but it is what they become by it. — John Ruskin

58. The more you train, the more you gain.

59. Live below your means.

60. You become the person you think you are.

61. Poverty is untested potential. — Denis Waitley

62. Does a cold beer really taste better at a fancy resort than it does in your backyard with close friends?

63. Always live on less money than you make. If you always pay yourself first, you create a lifelong savings plan.

64. It is human nature to want it and want it now; it is also a sign of immaturity. — Dave Ramsay

65. People should make their first investment in themselves. — Charles Schwab

66. Disciplined spending is investing today to reap benefits tomorrow.

67. Death is an opportunity not to be wasted.

68. It's not the years in your life that count; it's the life in your years. — Abraham Lincoln

69. Abundance creates the ability to give; giving creates more abundance. — Jim Stovall

70. Laughter is like internal jogging; it is a powerful antidote against stress.

71. If we fail to plan, we plan to fail.

72. Change your thoughts and you change your world. — Norman Vincent Peale

73. We need to replace doubts and fears with faith and confidence, and boredom with new habits, actions and skills.

74. If you don't like something, change it. If you can't change it, change your attitude. — Maya Angelou

75. Pain in life is inevitable, but suffering is optional.

76. Self-discipline's most valuable by-product is self-worth.

77. Worry is a down payment on a problem you may never have. — Joyce Meyer

78. We can worry ourselves to death, but we will never worry ourselves into a longer life.

79. Depression has been said to be anger turned inward.

80. Anything we believe we have to hide and cannot share has power over us.

81. Gratitude changes our attitude.

82. You are responsible for you. Life is truly a do-it-yourself project.

83. If nothing changes, nothing changes.

84. A choice to do nothing is still a choice.

85. Don't ask for life to be made easier; ask to be made better and stronger.

86. When we procrastinate, we don't avoid the pain; we just defer it.

87. An "I can do this" attitude will propel you into a world of new possibilities.

88. Be "obedient to the unenforceable." Accountability is actually a form of protection that guards us from painful consequences.

89. Good, better, best, never let it rest 'til your good is better and your better is best. — Children's nursery rhyme

90. Don't die with your music still inside you.

91. A great deal of talent is lost in this world for want of a little courage. — Sydney Smith

92. Twenty years from now you will be more disappointed by the things you didn't do than by the ones you did do. — Mark Twain.

93. The depth of our desire impacts the swiftness of our progress.

94. Every day, in every way, I am getting better and better!

RESOURCES

The following resources are by no means a comprehensive list of all that are available for the issues covered in the book; however, they do provide excellent sources to begin your quest for further information and help.

Abuse and Violence

- Abuse Help Center (United States):
  www.hclpguide.org/topics/abuse.htm
- Health Canada: Violence and Abuse:
  www.hc-sc.gc.ca/hc-ps/violence/index-eng.php
- The Hotline: National Domestic Violence Hotline (Canada):
  www.thehotline.org

Addictions

- Al-Anon Family Groups (for friends and families of problem drinkers) (International):
  www.al-anon.alateen.org

- Alcoholics Anonymous (World Services):
  www.aa.org

- Centre for Addiction and Mental Health (CAMH) (Toronto, Canada):
  www.camh.net

- Gamblers Anonymous (Unites States):
  www.gamblersanonymous.org

- Nar-Anon Family Groups (for friends and families of drug addicts) (World Services):
  www.nar-anon.org

- Narcotics Anonymous (World Services):
  www.na.org

- Overcomers Outreach (for addictions of all kinds):
  www.overcomersoutreach.org

- Overeaters Anonymous (International):
  www.oa.org

- Recovering Couples (World Services):
  www.recovering-couples.org

- S-Anon (for family and friends of sexalcholics) (International):
  www.sanon.org

- Sex Addicts Anonymous (International):
  www.sexaa.org

- Workaholics Anonymous (International):
  www.workaholics-anonymous.org

Conflict

- Thomas Kilmann Conflict Mode Instrument (TKI)
  www.kilmanndiagnostics.com/catalog/thomas-kilmann-
  conflict-mode-instrument

Donating Blood

- Canadian Blood Services:
  www.bloodservices.ca
- United Blood Services (United States):
  www.unitedbloodservices.org

Donating Organs and Tissues

- Donate Life America (United States):
  www.donatelife.net
- Living Donors Online (International Association of Living
  Organ Donors):
  www.livingdonorsonline.org
- Trillium Gift of Life Network (Canada):
  www.giftoflife.on.ca
- U.S. Department of Health and Human Services (government
  information on organ and tissue donation and transplantation):
  www.organdonor.gov

Gift Giving through Your Will and Estate Planning

- Community Foundations of Canada:
  www.cfc-fcc.ca
- Community Foundations (United States)
  www.communityfoundations.net

- Leave a Legacy (Canada):
  www.leavealegacy.ca
- Leave a Legacy (United States):
  www.leavealegacy.org

Government Revenue Agencies

- Canada Revenue Agency (CRA):
  www.cra-arc.gc.ca
- United States Internal Revenue Service (IRS):
  www.irs.gov

Hospice and Palliative Care

- Canadian Hospice Palliative Care Association:
  www.chpca.net
- National Hospice and Palliative Care Organization
  (United States):
  www.nhpco.org

Mental Health

- Canadian Mental Health Association:
  www.cmha.ca
- Mental Health America (United States):
  www.nmha.org
- National Institute of Mental Health (United States):
  www.nimh.nih.gov

Personality Testing

- Human Metrics (for a variety of personality tests):
  www.humanmetrics.com

- Myers & Briggs Foundation (for information on the Myers-Briggs Type Indicator (MBTI) personality assessment questionnaire):
  www.myersbriggs.org

- True Colors International (for information on the True Colors personality assessment tool):
  www.true-colors.com

Appendix IV

THE "I" STATEMENT EXERCISE

To complete the "I" Statement exercise, read the affirmations; there are ten "I" statements within each of the six components. As you read each statement, think how it applies to your life. Ask, "How satisfied am I with this aspect of my life?" or "How am I doing in regards to this statement?" Rate your answer on a scale from one to ten, with one representing no satisfaction and ten representing very satisfied.

FAITH: In yourself, in others, in life processes and in a higher spirit	
1. I believe in myself, trust myself and like the person I am.	1 2 3 4 5 6 7 8 9 10
2. I welcome change and know things work themselves out.	1 2 3 4 5 6 7 8 9 10
3. I practice self-discipline and self-control.	1 2 3 4 5 6 7 8 9 10
4. I trust the people in my life.	1 2 3 4 5 6 7 8 9 10

5. I am a positive person.	1 2 3 4 5 6 7 8 9 10
6. I have a dream and goals I am working toward.	1 2 3 4 5 6 7 8 9 10
7. I trust the process of life.	1 2 3 4 5 6 7 8 9 10
8. I know my beliefs affect the choices I make in a positive way.	1 2 3 4 5 6 7 8 9 10
9. I have a spiritual component to my life.	1 2 3 4 5 6 7 8 9 10
10. I do something every day to help me become a better person.	1 2 3 4 5 6 7 8 9 10

FAMILY: Your family of origin, immediate family and/or chosen family	
11. I enjoy time with all my family members.	1 2 3 4 5 6 7 8 9 10
12. I know how to set boundaries in family relationships.	1 2 3 4 5 6 7 8 9 10
13. I teach my children to be self-sufficient and of good character.	1 2 3 4 5 6 7 8 9 10
14. I offer praise regularly to family members.	1 2 3 4 5 6 7 8 9 10
15. I feel accepted and loved by my family members.	1 2 3 4 5 6 7 8 9 10
16. I communicate well with my family members.	1 2 3 4 5 6 7 8 9 10
17. I am committed to playing an active role in the lives of the children in my life.	1 2 3 4 5 6 7 8 9 10
18. I spend quality time with my partner at least twice a week.	1 2 3 4 5 6 7 8 9 10

19. I allow family members to see my vulnerabilities.	1 2 3 4 5 6 7 8 9 10
20. I show my family members that I love them unconditionally.	1 2 3 4 5 6 7 8 9 10

FITNESS: Your level of physical, nutritional, environmental, mental, emotional and spiritual fitness	
21. I am physically active a minimum of thirty minutes three times a week.	1 2 3 4 5 6 7 8 9 10
22. I am involved in creative work, studies or activities consistent with my values.	1 2 3 4 5 6 7 8 9 10
23. I regularly participate in a spiritual practice.	1 2 3 4 5 6 7 8 9 10
24. I manage my time effectively.	1 2 3 4 5 6 7 8 9 10
25. I spend time outdoors appreciating nature.	1 2 3 4 5 6 7 8 9 10
26. I limit my intake of alcohol, nicotine and drugs.	1 2 3 4 5 6 7 8 9 10
27. I set healthful limits for the amount of Internet, social media and TV I engage in.	1 2 3 4 5 6 7 8 9 10
28. I routinely get seven to eight hours of sleep a night.	1 2 3 4 5 6 7 8 9 10
29. I eat five to seven servings of fresh fruits and vegetables every day.	1 2 3 4 5 6 7 8 9 10
30. I understand my feelings and respond to them appropriately.	1 2 3 4 5 6 7 8 9 10

FRIENDS: Your buddies and those with whom you work and volunteer	
31. I have one or more close friends.	1 2 3 4 5 6 7 8 9 10
32. I am involved in service or volunteer work.	1 2 3 4 5 6 7 8 9 10
33. I enjoy the people I meet.	1 2 3 4 5 6 7 8 9 10
34. I know how to be my own best friend.	1 2 3 4 5 6 7 8 9 10
35. I enjoy a satisfying social life.	1 2 3 4 5 6 7 8 9 10
36. I have friends who respect my values.	1 2 3 4 5 6 7 8 9 10
37. I know how to set boundaries with my friends.	1 2 3 4 5 6 7 8 9 10
38. I offer help and assistance to others.	1 2 3 4 5 6 7 8 9 10
39. I handle conflict with others in a healthful manner.	1 2 3 4 5 6 7 8 9 10
40. I enjoy the work I do.	1 2 3 4 5 6 7 8 9 10

FINANCE: Your relationship with money—how much is enough and how to get it, keep it safe, grow it, have fun with it and give it away	
41. I earn the money I need to meet my financial obligations.	1 2 3 4 5 6 7 8 9 10
42. I earn the money I believe I deserve.	1 2 3 4 5 6 7 8 9 10
43. I spend money on what I need rather than on what I want.	1 2 3 4 5 6 7 8 9 10
44. I have financial assets/equity to build on.	1 2 3 4 5 6 7 8 9 10
45. I have a savings and investment plan I follow and review regularly.	1 2 3 4 5 6 7 8 9 10
46. I ask for help to plan my financial future.	1 2 3 4 5 6 7 8 9 10

47. I have an up-to-date will.	1 2 3 4 5 6 7 8 9 10
48. I donate money to a charitable cause I believe in.	1 2 3 4 5 6 7 8 9 10
49. I teach and encourage my children to earn and wisely manage their own money.	1 2 3 4 5 6 7 8 9 10
50. I take time to enjoy and have fun with some of the money I earn.	1 2 3 4 5 6 7 8 9 10

FUN: Your attitudes, choices, values and principles and how they impact the fun in your life	
51. I know how to say and use the word *no*.	1 2 3 4 5 6 7 8 9 10
52. I have respect for and abide by the law.	1 2 3 4 5 6 7 8 9 10
53. I laugh easily and regularly take part in fun and enjoyable activities.	1 2 3 4 5 6 7 8 9 10
54. I have someone to whom I stay accountable.	1 2 3 4 5 6 7 8 9 10
55. I look honestly at myself and admit to my foibles and weaknesses.	1 2 3 4 5 6 7 8 9 10
56. I seek advice and support from others.	1 2 3 4 5 6 7 8 9 10
57. I forgive myself and others.	1 2 3 4 5 6 7 8 9 10
58. I make wise choices according to my values and principles.	1 2 3 4 5 6 7 8 9 10
59. I am grateful for all I have in my life.	1 2 3 4 5 6 7 8 9 10
60. I strive for peace and calmness of mind.	1 2 3 4 5 6 7 8 9 10

THE BALANCE WHEEL OF HEALTH AND WELL-BEING EXERCISE

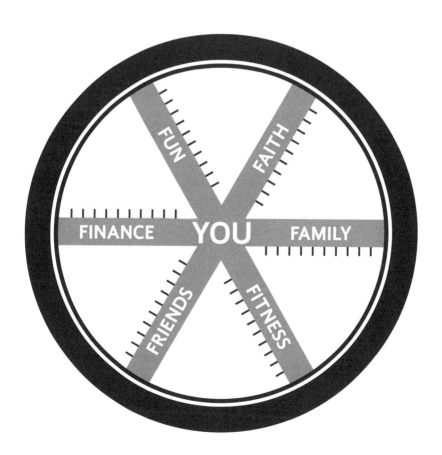

The balance wheel of health and well-being provides a visual representation of your level of satisfaction with your life and is an indicator of where there may be stress.

To complete this exercise, place an *X* on the spot best representing your present level of satisfaction with the specific spoke of the wheel. Use a scale of one to ten. The base of each spoke represents a low level of satisfaction, whereas the outer end represents a high level of satisfaction. There is no right or wrong. After you have marked each component, connect the *X*'s on each spoke. Look at the wheel and ask yourself these questions:

1. Can my wheel roll smoothly?
2. Am I completely deflated and riding on the rim?
3. What component needs to be reinflated?

SELECTED BIBLIOGRAPHY

This bibliography is by no means a complete record of all the sources I have consulted in the making of this book. Rather, it indicates the range of reading upon which I formed my ideas, and it serves as a list of works that I recommend if you wish to pursue any of the topics of this book in more detail.

Al-Anon Family Groups. *Courage to Change: One Day at a Time.* Virginia Beach, VA: Al-Anon Family Group Headquarters, 1992.

———. *Hope for Today.* Virginia Beach, VA: Al-Anon Family Group Headquarters, 2002.

———. *One Day at a Time.* New York: Al-Anon Family Group Headquarters, 1983.

———. *Opening Our Hearts: Transforming Our Losses.* Virginia Beach, VA: Al-Anon Family Group Headquarters, 2007.

Allen, James. *As a Man Thinketh.* Bellevue, WA: Emptitude Books, 2009.

Allen, Mark. *Happiness: One Day at a Time.* New York: Modus Vivendi, 1998.

———. *Love: One Day at a Time.* New York: Modus Vivendi, 1998.

———. *Success: One Day at a Time.* New York: Modus Vivendi, 1998.

Armstrong, Karen. *Twelve Steps to a Compassionate Life.* New York: Alfred A. Knopf, 2010.

Bach, David. *Smart Women Finish Rich: 9 Steps to Creating a Rich Future* (Canadian edition). Toronto, ON: Doubleday Canada, 2003.

———. *Smart Couples Finish Rich: 9 Steps to Creating a Rich Future for You and Your Partner* (Canadian edition). Toronto, ON: Doubleday Canada, 2003.

Barnett, Matthew. *The Cause within You: Finding the One Great Thing You Were Created to Do in This World.* With George Barna. Carol Stream, IL: BarnaBooks, 2011.

Beaulieu, John K. *Is Your Home a Healthy Home? How Common Household Chemicals May Gradually Be Making You and Your Family Sick.* Littleton, CO: RM Barry Publications, 2002.

Bell, Nicole, Eileen Conroy, Kim Wheatley, Benny Michaud, Candace Maracle, Jocelyne Pelletier, Barbara Filion, and Bernena Johnson. *The Ways of Knowing Guide.* Toronto, ON: Toronto Zoo and Turtle Island Conservation Programme, 2010.

Bonanno, George A. *The Other Side of Sadness: What the New Science of Bereavement Tells Us about Life after Loss.* New York: Basic Books, 2009.

Bradshaw, John. *Homecoming: Reclaiming and Championing Your Inner Child.* New York: Bantam Books, 1990.

Buckman, Robert. *I Don't Know What to Say: How to Help and Support Someone Who Is Dying.* Toronto, ON: Key Porter Books, 1988.

Buresh, Bernice, and Suzanne Gordon. *From Silence to Voice: What Nurses Know and Must Communicate to the Public.* 2nd ed. Ithaca, NY: Cornell University Press, 2006.

Carson, Rick. *Taming Your Gremlins: A Surprisingly Simple Method for Getting Out of Your Own Way.* New York: HarperCollins, 2003.

Chapman, Gary D. *The Five Love Languages: How to Express Heartfelt Commitment to Your Mate.* Chicago: Northfield Publishing, 2004.

————. *The World's Easiest Guide to Family Relationships*. With Randy Southern. Chicago: Northfield Publishing, 2001.

Clason, George S. *The Richest Man in Babylon*. New York: Signet, 1988.

Cloud, Henry, and John Townsend. *Boundaries: When to Say Yes, When to Say No to Take Control of Your Life*. Grand Rapids, MI: Zondervan, 2001.

Covey, Stephen R. *The 7 Habits of Highly Effective People: Powerful Lessons in Personal Change*. New York: Free Press, 2004.

————. *The Speed of Trust: The One Thing That Changes Everything*. New York: Free Press, 2006.

Crowley, Chris, and Henry S. Lodge. *Younger Next Year: Live Strong, Fit and Sexy—Until You're 80 and Beyond*. New York: Workman Publishing, 2007.

Daly, Melissa. "How Healthy Are Your Friendships?" *Prevention*, May 2011.

Deans, Thomas William. *Every Family's Business: 12 Common Sense Questions to Protect Your Wealth*. Orangeville, ON: Détente Financial Press, 2009.

Eggerichs, Emerson. *Love and Respect for a Lifetime*. Nashville, TN: Thomas Nelson, 2010.

Exline, Eric. *The Healthy Cell Concept*. Nampa, ID: AIM International, 1995.

Freston, Kathy. *Quantum Wellness: A Practical and Spiritual Guide to Health and Happiness*. New York: Weinstein Books, 2008.

Gaber, Christine, and Charlene Day. *Why Do I Feel This Way? Cutting through the Health Confusion*. Caledon East, ON: Health through Knowledge, 2009.

Goleman, Daniel. *Emotional Intelligence: Why It Can Matter More than IQ*. New York: Bantam Books, 1997.

Gray, John. *Men Are from Mars, Women Are from Venus: The Classic Guide to Understanding*. New York: HarperCollins, 1992.

Haas, Elson M. *Staying Healthy with Nutrition: The Complete Guide to Diet and Nutritional Medicine.* Berkeley, CA: Celestial Arts, 2006.

Hill, Napoleon. *Think and Grow Rich.* Valparaiso, IN: Life Success Group, 2009.

Jamal, Azim, and Harvey McKinnon. *The Power of Giving: Creating Abundance in Your Home, at Work, and in Your Community.* Nashville, TN: Hushion House Publishing, 2005.

James, Dawn. *Raise Your Vibration, Transform Your Life: A Practical Guide for Attaining Better Health, Vitality and Inner Peace.* Uxbridge, ON: Lotus Moon Press, 2010.

Kaspardlov, Dessa. *The Fireman and the Waitress: The True Story of an Ordinary Couple Reaching Extraordinary Heights.* Ontario, Canada: Dessaco, 2009.

Keirsey, David, and Marilyn Bates. *Please Understand Me: Character and Temperament Types.* 5th ed. Del Mar, CA: Prometheus Nemesis Book Company, 1984.

Kent, Graeme. *Things to Do Now That You're 60.* London, UK: MQ Publications, 2005.

Thomas, Kenneth Wayne, and Ralph H. Kilmann. *Thomas-Kilmann Conflict Mode Instrument.* Mountain View, CA: CPP Inc., 2002.

Kubassek, Ben. *Achieving Real Balance: How to Succeed without Burnout.* Renfrew, ON: Creative Bound, 2002. Audiobook.

Kübler-Ross, Elisabeth. *Death: The Final Stage of Growth.* New York: Simon & Schuster, 1975.

———. *On Death and Dying: What the Dying Have to Teach Doctors, Nurses, Clergy, and Their Own Families.* New York: Simon & Schuster, 1969.

Kuhl, David. *What Dying People Want: Practical Wisdom for the End of Life.* Toronto, ON: Anchor Canada, 2003.

Kurzweil, Raymond. *The Age of Intelligent Machines.* Boston, MA: MIT Press, 1999.

Langemeier, Loral. *Building Your Wealth Cycles*. Live Out Loud, 2003. Audiobook, 6 compact discs.

———. *The Millionaire Maker: Act, Think, and Make Money the Way the Wealthy Do*. New York: McGraw-Hill, 2006.

———. *The Millionaire Maker's Guide to Wealth Cycle Investing*. New York: McGraw-Hill, 2007.

Lawson, Douglas M. *More Give to Live: How Giving Can Change Your Life*. San Diego, CA: Alti Publishing, 1997.

Leaf, Caroline. *Who Switched Off My Brain? Controlling Toxic Thoughts and Emotions*. Southlake, TX: Thomas Nelson, 2009.

Levin, Jeff. *God, Faith, and Health: Exploring the Spirituality-Healing Connection*. New York: John Wiley & Sons, 2001.

Lipton, Bruce. *The Biology of Belief: Unleashing the Power of Consciousness, Matter & Miracles*. Santa Rosa, CA: Elite Books, 2005.

Loomans, Diana, and Karen Kohlberg. *The Laughing Classroom: Everyone's Guide to Teaching with Humor and Play*. Tiburon, CA: H. J. Kramer, 2002.

Lowe, Janet. *The Super Saver: Fundamental Strategies for Building Wealth*. Lafayette, LA: Longman Financial Services Publishing, 1990.

Lupien, Sonia. *Well Stressed: Manage Stress Before It Turns Toxic*. Mississauga, ON: John Wiley & Sons, 2012.

MacArthur, John. *Anxious for Nothing: God's Cure for the Cares of Your Soul*. Colorado Springs, CO: David C. Cook, 2012.

MacKenzie, Warren. "How to Be Financially Secure on a Tight Budget." *Home Digest*, West Edition, Early Spring, 2011, 23.

Maslow, Abraham H. *The Maslow Business Reader*. Edited by Deborah C. Stevens. Hoboken, NJ: John Wiley & Sons, 2000.

———. *Religions, Values, and Peak-Experiences*. New York: Penguin Arkana, 1994.

———. *Toward a Psychology of Being*. 3rd ed. Hoboken, NJ: John Wiley & Sons, 1998.

Maté, Gabor. *When the Body Says No: Understanding the Stress-Disease Connection.* Hoboken, NJ: John Wiley & Sons, 2003.

Merton, Thomas. *No Man Is an Island.* Orlando, FL; Harcourt, 1983.

Meyer, Joyce. *100 Ways to Simplify Your Life.* New York: FaithWords, 2008.

———. *Battlefield of the Mind: Winning the Battle in Your Mind.* New York: FaithWords, 2002.

———. *Eat the Cookie … Buy the Shoes: Giving Yourself Permission to Lighten Up.* New York: FaithWords, 2010.

———. *Hearing from God Each Morning: 365 Daily Devotions.* New York: FaithWords, 2010.

———. *Living Beyond Your Feelings: Controlling Emotions So They Don't Control You.* New York: FaithWords, 2011.

———. *Never Give Up! Relentless Determination to Overcome Life's Challenges.* New York: FaithWords, 2008.

———. *Power Thoughts: 12 Strategies to Win the Battle of the Mind.* New York: FaithWords, 2010.

Moritz, Andreas. *Cancer Is Not a Disease, It's a Survival Mechanism.* Landrum, SC: Ener-Chi, 2008.

Myss, Caroline. *Anatomy of the Spirit: The Seven Stages of Power and Healing.* New York: Three Rivers Press, 1996.

———. *Why People Don't Heal and How They Can.* New York: Three Rivers Press, 1997.

Patchell-Evans, David. *Living the Good Life: Your Guide to Health and Success.* Toronto, ON: ECW Press, 2004.

Peale, Norman Vincent. *The Power of Positive Thinking.* New York: Ballantine Books, 1996.

Peck, M. Scott. *The Road Less Traveled: A New Psychology of Love, Traditional Values and Spiritual Growth.* 2nd ed. New York: Touchstone, 1998.

Pert, Candace B. *Molecules of Emotion: Why You Feel the Way You Feel.* New York: Touchstone, 1999.

Poe, Richard. *The Wave 3 Way to Building Your Downline.* Roseville, CA: Prima Lifestyles, 1997.

Ponder, Catherine. *The Dynamic Laws of Prayer.* 2nd revised ed. Camarillo, CA: DeVorss & Company, 1987.

Ramsay, David. *The Total Money Makeover: A Proven Plan for Financial Fitness.* Nashville, TN: Thomas Nelson, 2003.

Robbins, Anthony. *Get the Edge: A 7-Day Program to Transform Your Life.* San Diego, CA: The Anthony Robins Companies, 2001. Audiobook set.

Rohn, Jim. *The Art of Exceptional Living.* Niles, IL: Nightingale-Conant Corporation, 2003. Audiobook set.

Schaef, Anne Wilson. *Meditations for Living in Balance: Daily Solutions for People Who Do Too Much.* New York: HarperCollins, 2000.

Schwab, Charles. *Charles Schwab's Guide to Financial Independence: Simple Solutions for Busy People.* New York: Three Rivers Press, 1998.

Schwartz, David J. *The Magic of Thinking Big.* New York: Simon & Schuster, 1987.

Selye, Hans. *Stress in Health and Disease.* Waltham, MA: Butterworth-Heinemann, 1976.

———. *The Stress of Life.* Revised ed. Whitby, ON: McGraw-Hill, 1978.

———. *Stress Without Distress: How to Use Stress as a Positive Force to Achieve a Rewarding Lifestyle.* New York: Penguin Books, 1975.

Shakespeare, William. *William Shakespeare: The Complete Works.* New York: Dorset Press, 1988.

Shalof, Tilda. *A Nurse's Story: Life, Death and In-between in an Intensive Care Unit.* Toronto, ON: McClelland & Stewart, 2004.

———. *The Making of a Nurse.* Toronto, ON: McClelland & Stewart, 2008.

Siebold, Steve. *How Rich People Think.* London, UK: London House Press, 2010.

Skloot, Rebecca. *The Immortal Life of Henrietta Lacks*. New York: Crown Publishers, 2010.

Springhouse. *Pathophysiology Made Incredibly Easy!* 4th ed. Ambler, PA: Lippincott Williams & Wilkins, 2008.

Stanley, Charles. *Success God's Way*. Markham, ON: In Touch Ministries, 2003. Audiobook set.

Stanley, Thomas J. *Stop Acting Rich ... and Start Living Like a Real Millionaire*. Hoboken, NJ: John Wiley & Sons, 2009.

Stanley, Thomas J., and William D. Danko. *The Millionaire Next Door*. New York: Simon & Schuster, 1996.

Stovall, Jim. *The Ultimate Gift*. Colorado Springs, CO: David C. Cook, 2001.

Swindoll, Charles R. *You and Your Money*. Piano, TX: IFL Publishing House, 2011.

Vaz-Oxlade, Gail. *Debt-free Forever: Take Control of Your Money and Your Life*. New York: The Experiment, 2010.

Visor, Sonya. *Who I've Become Is Not Who I Am*. Racine, WI: Covenant House Press, 2010.

Waitley, Denis, and Reni L. Witt. *The Joy of Working: The 30-Day System to Success, Wealth, and Happiness on the Job*. New York: Ballantine Books, 1995.

Warren, Rick. *The Purpose-Driven Life: What on Earth Am I Here For?* Grand Rapids, MI: Zondervan, 2002.

Weider, Marcia. *Making Your Dreams Come True*. New York: Harmony Books, 1999.

Wright, Nicholas Thomas. *Surprised by Hope: Rethinking Heaven, the Resurrection, and the Mission of the Church*. New York: HarperOne, 2008.

Ziglar, Zig. *Staying Up, Up, Up in a Down, Down World: Daily Hope for the Daily Grind*. Carol Stream, IL: Oasis Audio, 2004. Audiobook set.

———. *Strategies for Success: Blueprint for Achievement*. Plano, TX: Ziglar Training Systems, 2006. Audiobook set.

INDEX